IN SEARCH OF THE GOOD LIFE

IN SEARCH OF THE GOOD LIFE

Emmanuel Levinas, Psychoanalysis, and the Art of Living

Paul Marcus

Routledge
Taylor & Francis Group
LONDON AND NEW YORK

First published 2010 by Karnac Books Ltd.

Published 2019 by Routledge
2 Park Square, Milton Park, Abingdon, Oxon OX14 4RN
52 Vanderbilt Avenue, New York, NY 10017

First issued in hardback 2019

Routledge is an imprint of the Taylor & Francis Group, an informa business

British Library Cataloguing in Publication Data

A C.I.P. for this book is available from the British Library

ISBN 13: 978-0-367-10644-7 (hbk)
ISBN 13: 978-1-85575-723-3 (pbk)

Edited, designed and produced by The Studio Publishing Services Ltd
www.publishingservicesuk.co.uk
e-mail: studio@publishingservicesuk.co.uk

CONTENTS

ACKNOWLEDGEMENTS

I wish to thank my colleague and good friend William B. Helmreich, Professor of Sociology and Judaic Studies, for his helpful critical comments about my entire manuscript. My editor, Morris Rabinowitz, as always, helped make my manuscript read much more clearly and thoughtfully. Thanks also go to my wife Irene, a child and adult psychoanalyst, who not only read every word of my manuscript a few times, but graciously endured a husband who was often upstairs in his room writing while she kept everything else in our household going smoothly. Finally, I am grateful to my children, Raphael and Gabriela, whose inquiring minds gave me further impetus to write this book.

"For I believe that no man, however enlightened and holy he is, can ever arrive until the others, *all* the others, have started out to follow him . . . We never climb alone, though we often seem to do so."

Gabriel Marcel

ABOUT THE AUTHOR

Paul Marcus, PhD, is a supervising and training analyst at the National Psychological Association for Psychoanalysis. He is the author of *Being for The Other, Emmanuel Levinas, Ethical Living and Psychoanalysis; Autonomy in the Extreme Situation: Bruno Bettelheim, the Nazi Concentration Camps, and the Mass Society; Ancient Religious Wisdom, Spirituality and Psychoanalysis,* among other books. Dr Marcus is married and has two children. He lives in Great Neck, New York, and can be reached at Tibs9@aol.com.

To Dr Philip M. Stone
In gratitude

Introduction: Levinas, psychoanalysis, and the art of living the good life

"The only morality is therefore one of kindness"

Emmanuel Levinas

Emmanuel Levinas (1906–1995), French phenomenological philosopher and Talmudic commentator, is regarded as perhaps the greatest ethical philosopher of our time. Jacques Derrida, the founder of deconstruction and himself an illustrious philosopher, for example, wrote, "the reverberations of his thought will have changed the course of philosophical reflection in our time, and of our reflection on philosophy" (Derrida, 1999, p. 4). While Levinas enjoys prominence in the philosophical and scholarly community, especially in Europe, there are few, if any, books or articles written that take Levinas's extremely difficult to understand, if not obtuse, philosophy and apply it to the everyday lives of "real" people struggling to give greater meaning and purpose, especially ethical meaning, to their personal lives. This book attempts to fill the large gap in the Levinas literature, mainly through using a Levinasian-inspired, ethically-infused psychoanalytic approach, an approach that I first developed in *Being For The Other: Emmanuel Levinas, Ethical Living and Psychoanalysis* (2008). I aim to suggest how Levinas's ethical insights into the personal, the interpersonal, and human flourishing (i.e., creative, life-affirming living), when merged with a psychoanalytic sensibility, can widen and deepen our capacity to live more ethically, more "for the Other", in our everyday personal lives. All of the essays included in this book are animated by the Levinasian assumption that it is the ethical relation to the other person (and, in one case, dog!) that is primary. That is, there is a human tendency in us, an often inhibited, muted, or repressed tendency, as psychoanalysts have taught us, to see the needs of others as more important (or at least as important as) than our own and therefore be willing to sacrifice for others. Moreover, once this human tendency to be for the Other is consciously embraced and made part of one's way of being in the world, the possibility for a greater degree of personal fulfilment and happiness is often enhanced. Thus, the art of living the "good life", as I call it, involves embracing "goodness" as one's guiding metaphor, an existential orientation in which, says Levinas, "the Other counts more than myself" (1969, p. 247). As social psychologists have repeatedly shown, in social life, paradoxically, it is often the case that "the more you give, the more you get". Being for the Other, in other words, is often self-affirming.

In order to further contextualize the focus of this book, it is important for the reader to get a sense of how I conceive of psychoanalysis, how I situate Levinas as a thinker and how I "read" him. Most important, the reader needs to comprehend the way in which I merge Levinas and psychoanalysis into a "Levinasian-inspired, ethically-infused psychoanalysis," an approach that strives to illuminate those ethical aspects of our common psychological and social experiences that are usually neglected in conventional psychological and psychoanalytic renderings. Moreover, such an approach points to the self-enhancing aspects of embracing a wider and deeper ethical way of being in one's personal life, ethics here defined, most simply, as responsibility for the Other, often before oneself.

Defining psychoanalysis

I conceive of psychoanalysis as a form of life, a resource for individuals who can appropriate the life- and identity-defining narrative of psychoanalysis when they seek to understand, endure, and, possibly, conquer the problems that beset the human condition: despair, loss, tragedy, anxiety, and conflict. In effect, they try to synthesize, come to grips with, the emotionally painful experiences of life through a psychoanalytic outlook. In other words, psychoanalysis can be viewed as what Foucault called a "technology of the self . . . an exercise of the self, by which one attempts to develop and transform oneself, and to attain a certain mode of being" (Foucault, 1989, p. 433). As philosopher Pierre Hadot noted in another context, psychoanalysis can be understood as a "spiritual exercise", a tool for living life correctly. The aim of a spiritual exercise is to foster a deep modification of the individual's way of "seeing and being", a decisive change in how he lives his practical, everyday life (Hadot, 1997, p. 83). According to this view, playing off the words of Levinas, psychoanalysis is "a difficult wisdom concerned with truths that correlate to virtues": in other words, it is a powerful tool for the art of living the "good life" (Levinas, 1989a, p. 275).

Situating Levinas in philosophy

In this book, Levinas is "read" as one of the many philosophers interested less in striving for wisdom, but more in trying to influence the way people live their lives. In other words, Levinas does not start off with a traditional conception of philosophy, but, like that of some of the ancient philosophers and Talmudic rabbis, his discourse is best conceived as a tool to facilitate the striving for self-transformation and self-transcendence. His implied goal was to transform his readers and to provoke them into changing their manner of living, towards greater ethical thinking, feeling, and, most importantly, acting. For me, Levinas is most usefully read as a philosopher who concentrated on shaping the souls of individual readers to help them to become better people, people more capable of being for the Other before being for oneself. As Levinas noted, more than ethics, he was interested in "holiness": "You know, they often speak of ethics to describe what I do, but what interests me when all is said and done is not ethics, it is the holy, the holiness of the holy" (Derrida, 1999, p. 4). This holiness occurs when the concern for the other, his reasonable material, psychological, and spiritual needs, takes precedence over the self (e.g., raising children, at its best). It is through a Levinasian sensibility merged with the best of psychoanalytic insight that self-transformation toward autonomy can take place, and its therapeutic and edifying impact on one's ethical life can be set in motion. Levinas, in other words, can be situated and read in the company of those great thinkers, certain ancient philosophers, and Nietzsche, who regard philosophy as a way of working on oneself, as "a way of life" or "soul care". I believe that Levinas was advocating the need for a radical reconfiguration of self-identity, radical changes in character structure, and values and beliefs that make being for the Other before being for oneself seem "natural", or almost "natural".

A Levinasian-inspired, ethically-infused psychoanalysis

As I have said, though Levinas is regarded by many philosophers as possibly the greatest ethicist of the past century, he is hardly known by most mainstream psychoanalysts. Levinas's philosophy, at least as I interpret it (Marcus, 2008), provides the basis for the development of a new psychoanalytic "master narrative" (a theory of the human condition that guides its clinical practice), one that makes the ethical demand of the Other the ultimate affect-integrating, meaning-making, and action-guiding hermeneutic horizon. Indeed, such a Levinasian-inspired, ethically-infused psychoanalysis radically disrupts, undermines, and challenges our usual psychoanalytic way of thinking about ourselves and our analysands; it suggests that the main goal of analysis is helping the analysand awaken "to a moral life" that is conterminous "with the discovery that the Other is the first to be respected, served" (Peperzak, 1993, p. 111) and tended to, before oneself. It is the development of a moral consciousness, defined as the mindfulness "of the privilege the other has relative to me" (ibid., p. 112) that characterizes a successful analysis.

Though all of the current master narratives—man as pleasure seeking (e.g., Freud), object seeking (e.g., Klein and Fairbairn), and meaning seeking (e.g., Schaefer and Spence), for example—have great appeal and usefulness (Weinstein, 1990, p. 27), I am suggesting that the analytic community consider an alternative paradigm in its theorizing, one that is rooted in the evocative Levinasian perspective on existence: the sacrificing mother "who takes bread from her mouth and the milk from her body to give to . . . [her] child" (Kunz, 1998, p. 148). The powerful story of a mother and child in Turkey who were trapped under the earthquake rubble for days comes to mind. When her child became weak from loss of nourishing fluids, the woman cut the tip of her finger with a piece of broken glass for the child to suck her blood. Remarkably, they both survived (ibid.). Such a Levinasian-inspired narrative of the human condition points psychoanalysis in a very different direction than is conventionally conceived. It emphasizes, according to Davis (1996, p. 54), that "the responsibility for, and obligation to, the Other are absolute". They are greater than the individual's responsibility to satisfy them, there is always more demanded, and they are never fulfilled by any single deed. In other words, "as a moral subject", the individual is always found lacking, because ethics is not just a component of one's existence as psychoanalysis usually assumes, it delimits the entire realm in which one resides. Such a notion of the subject, constituted by the encounter with the Other, "the basis of ethical relations founded on the encounter" (ibid., p. 79), suggests a reorientation for psychoanalysis in at least one fundamental way, towards a psychoanalysis that moves away from viewing the Other as primarily a source of gratification of one's relational needs for companionship, friendship, love, and intimacy. Rather, following Levinas, I am imagining a psychoanalytic subject that lives with a very different sensibility, a very different way of being in the world, one in which he declares with the fullness of his being, like Abraham—"Hineni"—"Here I am!" Such a person, says Levinas, knows and feels with radical clarity and moral passion that "the node of the subjective is knotted in ethics understood as responsibility" (Levinas, 1985, p. 95). In my imaginings, this is a psychoanalytic subject that is less driven by pleasure, meaning, or even object seeking and attachment needs, as analysts usually use those terms. Rather, in this new psychoanalytic version of subjectivity, it is the image of the panic- and terror-stricken Turkish mother and her vulnerable, weak, near-death child who lay helplessly under the rubble from the earthquake that the Levinasian-inspired psychoanalytic subject is haunted by. Levinas's notion of subjectivity is thus conceptualized in strictly ethical terms, as responsibility for the Other, a "demand" or "commandment to giving and serving" (ibid., p. 119). The self, Levinas evocatively declares, is first and unrefusably "hostage" to the summoning Other, responsible even for what he has not done: guilt without fault. Moreover, it is important to note, Levinas's ethical subject does not augment a preceding existential base, as psychoanalysts usually assume in their various versions of subjectivity. Rather, the subject is, from the outset, the responsible self-hostage to the Other.

Thus, the central aim of this book is to apply a Levinasian-inspired, ethically-infused psychoanalysis to ordinary aspects of human experience, relating to a beloved pet, tending to a dying mother, raising children, using food as a way of self-transformation (e.g., vegetarianism), using gossip to navigate the intricacies of social interaction, for example, in order to suggest that our relation to ourselves, to others, and to social systems can become more ethical, more animated by responsibility for the Other. Perhaps, most importantly, I hope to bring Levinas's daunting ethical philosophy down to the level of where it actually "hits" the reader, "moves" him to feel, think, and act differently, more Other-directed and Other-regarding, while also being respectful of the complexity, profundity, and personal arduousness of Levinas's philosophy of living.

A word on the layout of the book

A cursory glance at the table of contents should give the reader a good sense of the themes of the book, all of which are concerned with common psychological and social experiences in our western culture. All of the chapters are broadly correlated with typical Levinasian themes and draw from my experiences as a practising psychoanalyst over the past twenty years, including, following Freud, drawing on my self-analysis and personal experience, as well as my work as a court-appointed forensic evaluator used in child custody and criminal matters. Although this book deals with "heavy" and complex Levinasian themes, I have tried very hard to limit the Levinasian and psychoanalytic jargon and to keep the references down to a minimum (to this aim, I added a short Levinasian glossary), so as not to distract the reader from feeling the

"Levinasian effect"; that is, from experiencing the depth, possibility, and beauty that come to mind and heart when imaginatively engaging the rhythm of Levinas's transfiguring ethical vision. As I hope to show, the art of living the "good life" entails just such a radical transforming of consciousness characterized by an upsurge of love, freedom, hope and joy. As Levinas said, "For every man, assuming responsibility for the Other is a way of testifying to the glory of the Infinite, and of being inspired" (Levinas, 1985, p. 113).

Paul Marcus
January 2010

CHAPTER ONE

"I'm just wild about Harry!" A psychoanalyst reflects on his relationship with his dog*

> "It really explains why we can love an animal . . . with such extraordinary intensity; affection without ambivalence, the simplicity of a life free from the almost unbearable conflict of civilization, the beauty of an existence complete in itself . . . Often when stroking Jo-fi [Freud's dog] I have caught myself humming a melody which, unmusical as I am, I can't help recognizing as the aria from *Don Giovanni*: 'a bond of friendship unites us both'"
>
> Sigmund Freud

Like Freud, and, for that matter, like any devoted dog owner you happen to meet on the street or in the park, I love my dog. "He is my best friend," I often say to people. Harry, a one-year-old Cocker Spaniel, was a "rescue" dog, a code word for a pup that was given up by his owner and either left on the street or given to a dogs' home. In Harry's case, he was abused and abandoned, a stray found on the Brooklyn side of the Belt Parkway, starving, filthy with fleas and tics, and very frightened. According

*An earlier version of this essay appeared in the *Psychoanalytic Review* (2007).

to the foster lady, Shirley, a remarkable woman from whom I obtained Harry and whose life mission is to rescue Cocker Spaniels from certain death on the street and find them a good home, Harry was a sweet dog, though a traumatized one. When we first met Harry in her Queens, New York home, he was still very skinny and fearful, with long floppy ears and sad eyes. Nevertheless, within a few minutes it was clear that both my wife and I, a child and adult psychoanalyst, respectively, felt a summoning call from Harry: "Help me, love me, take good care of me."

Pausing for a moment, and having wondered to ourselves out loud, "Are we crazy?", having just sent off our second of two children to college and having spent many of the preceding months fantasizing about how nice life would be without any children to look after (call it a neurotic decision to deal with our "empty nest" feelings), we nevertheless decided to adopt Harry. "Maybe we will get it right the third time," I joked to my wife! As this chapter testifies, our decision to take Harry home was stunningly right, as "The Pup", as we sometimes call him, has been a transformational living presence in our lives, one that has immeasurably enhanced us and inspired us to ask ourselves, why is this so?

This chapter aims to explore the nature of the relationship between a person and his dog. It attempts to delineate some of the reasons why dogs, and by extension other beloved pets ("companion animals", to be politically correct), have such a powerfully positive psychological meaning and effect on their owners. That is, I will describe some of the psychodynamics between an owner and his dog, as well as the developmental needs and wishes that the owner uniquely satisfies through his hound. Most importantly perhaps, following Levinas, I suggest that what makes one's relationship with an adored dog so moving, so self-transformational and self-transcendent, is that emanating from the hound, especially from his "face", there is an irresistible ethical call, an ethical address, of responsibility for the other. Indeed, in my case, Harry, experienced as unique, as an irreducible singularity, is a testimony to a kind of pure love, that is, he represents the gift of diffused love inseparable from my responsibility for him, and my moral obligation to him (Calin, 2005, pp. 73–74). In short, Harry has taught me how to love more deeply and selflessly, and for this I am most thankful. Martin Buber also movingly describes the "deeply stirring happening" in his childhood (he was eleven years old), while spending the summer on his grandparents' estate. There, the adult Buber says, he had an I–Thou encounter with "my darling, a broad dapple-grey horse". Stroking his "mighty mane", "what I experienced in touch with the animal was the Other, the immense otherness of the Other" (Buber, 1965, p. 23).

The context of obtaining Harry

In 2004, about 36% of American household included children; more than 60% included pet animals (Becker, 2006, p. 17). An equally astonishing fact is that one-third of dog owners would be willing to accept a 5% decrease in salary to be able to take their dogs to work, according to a recent survey (*The Boston Phoenix*, 30 June, 2006, p. 6). Moreover, as Grier points out in her recent historical study *Pets in America* (Grier, 2006), pet owners now typically describe their animals as their "best friends" or as "family members". In my case, as I have said, the acquisition of Harry was intimately connected with my family composition, or rather with the dramatic change in its configuration, both of my children having left home to go to university.

In an entirely obvious manner, Harry was a replacement child. That is, he satisfied some primordial need in my wife and me to continue to be in the parenting role: to provide nurturance, stability, and protection to a vulnerable being. Indeed, the replacement meaning of Harry for our children was evident in a variety of ways: in taking great care in feeding, exercising, and looking after Harry's physical well-being, especially early on when he was so skinny and physically fragile. Thus, as with my children when they were young, I made sure that Harry ate the best food (the expensive, organic Paul Newman dog food); that I took him for a run in the park or woods every day as opposed to a short functional walk around the block (to keep him strong, alert and happy); I routinely took Harry to the veterinarian and responsibly gave him the medicines he needed, closely monitoring his progress; I hugged, kissed, and played with him frequently and with great enthusiasm, telling him what a great dog he was; I tried to help him to get over his fearfulness, especially towards strangers, a skittishness that reflected the after-effects of having been beaten as a puppy. As we did when our children were infants, my wife and I frequently talk to Harry as if he understood us: "Sweetie pie, are you tired today?" "Darling, are you having fun playing with your soft toy?" Like both my children, Harry was a bad sleeper who would frequently come into our bed in the middle of the night, forcing me to get up and put him back in his own bed. As with my children, however, there were many nights when I was too tired or lazy to get up, or simply enjoyed his warm company, and Harry slept next to us. Perhaps the best examples indicating that the Harry–child analogy was operative was that I frequently referred to the veterinarian as the paediatrician, and a few times I called Harry by my son's name. Most poignantly, as with my three-year-old daughter, once when Harry accidentally ate some poisonous materials that required an emergency visit to the veterinarian, I remember cradling the half-conscious puppy and feeling the same kind of intense anxiety and worry about Harry's survival that I did for my sick daughter.

However, we had no ambitions for Harry, as we did for our children, when we brought him into our world. We did not fantasize that he would become a great diplomat who would solve the Middle East conflict (my son's choice of study), or a famous actress (my daughter's goal). Instead, Harry just had to keep being Harry: loveable. But why is Harry so loveable, and what does this have to do with my two children, who left home, never to return as the children they once were?

Unlike my children, Harry was fairly easy to please. In fact, not only did he not talk back, he was clearly grateful in his own way, and, perhaps most importantly, loyal. Harry would never choose to abandon me for another master, he would never say to himself, so to speak, "Hey Harry, the folks down the road serve better nosh", or "I can get more hugs and kisses elsewhere". No, as long as I feed him and take good care of him he will remain loyal to the end, never abandoning me. While my children pay lip service to a similar principle, like most parents, I do not entirely believe that they have the loyalty and devotion that Harry does, nor should they, of course, nor should I need or expect them to, either. In fact, I want my children to separate psychologically from us, get married, have children, productive careers, and live their lives as they want to in their own dwellings. For the most part, I envision my children having a background involvement in my life as I get older, while I never want Harry to separate and live elsewhere.

What I am getting at is that Harry satisfies a very basic need that I have, and, for that matter, seems to be a constituent part of the human condition: he blunts the horror of separation and abandonment that most of us somewhere feel deep down in our infantile selves and spend considerable conscious and unconscious psychic energy managing. He does this through his faithfulness, expressed by a thoroughly gratifying, affirming, and predictable set of behaviours. When I come home every night hungry, tired, and spent, I know for sure that Harry will respond to the doorbell the same adoring way he always does: he starts to bark loudly and frantically; I put my hand through the letter box and he jumps up and starts to feverishly lick it; I open the door and he jumps all over me, tail wagging, licking and kissing me, seemingly utterly thrilled that I have returned home. It is a greeting to die for! Compare this to my teenage children, who hardly notice that I have come home, and to my wife, who is dead tired from a long day of analytic work and, mainly out of politeness, just manages to say, "Hi, how was your day?" In other words, Harry provides an almost magical, though reliable, sense that one can separate from a loved one and return to him, with everything being as one left it—no, better.

Harry's greeting of me when I come home is a stark contrast to the way my teenage children greeted me, though that was not always the case. Indeed, when my children were younger, especially when they were toddlers, I recall a fairly high degree of excitement when I came home, though I could easily play second fiddle to a good Disney video they were watching. Actually, there is an important connection between Harry and toddlers, for, in my view, part of the secret of Harry's charm and lovability is that he is like a toddler in so many ways, without, however, the "terrible twos". Harry is playful, zestful, curious, cute, and affectionate. He is hardly oppositional, and when he is, it is usually for a good reason and entirely predictable, as when he does not want to have his leash put on when leaving the park. These moments are admittedly annoying, especially when it takes ten minutes to coax Harry to let me approach and leash him, requiring me to use the very skills that I use to engage patients who have similar approach–avoidance and "closeness" issues. Nevertheless, for some reason, these occasional difficulties leave no negative trace in me, probably because, unlike toddlers, Harry's resistance is not oppositional for its own sake. Such difficult moments with Harry are far outweighed by the fact that, like a toddler, he manifests "a love affair with the world", one that evokes in me an upsurge of joy similar to what I felt when my children were in that adorable stage of development.

"A bond of friendship unites us both"

As the epigraph to this chapter suggests, Freud thought that the secret to his uniquely strong attachment to his dog was that his relationship to Jo-fi embodied the highest form of friendship. What was Freud getting at when he made this provocative claim?

Freud, working from a largely Greek, specifically Aristotelian conception of human happiness, one that stressed "functioning well" in love and work as the gold standard (Wallwork, 2005, p. 287), did not write about the psychology of friendship in any systematic way. Thus, we have to piece together what his view of friendship was, in particular, by extrapolating from his Aristotelian-informed conception of the human condition. Only in this way will we be able to apprehend what Freud may have meant when he described Jo-fi as his uniquely esteemed friend that he loved "with such extraordinary intensity".

In Books VIII and IX of the *Nicomachean Ethics*, Aristotle briefly discusses three forms of friendships: friendships of pleasure, of utility, and of excellence. Each one of these forms of friendships is characterized by mutual affection between equals, with the differences between them mainly rooted in the different types of affectionate relatedness or friendliness involved. That is, they have their specific motivations, expectations, and trajectories that apply to human relations and, by analogy, to my relationship with Harry.

A friendship of pleasure is one in which two people simply enjoy one another's company, though what both parties mainly seek is their own pleasure and satisfaction. For Aristotle the "good" that is desired for both people is enjoyment, and relationships of this type tend to dissipate and end when what had given enjoyment stops doing so. In the case of my relationship with Harry, it is clear to me that Harry and I enjoy being together; everything from petting his soft, silky fur that both feels good and is comforting, to his toddler-like charm, actually his entire demeanour, is extremely pleasurable. Clearly, Harry feels likewise, or he would not seek me out to be stroked, sit by my feet, follow me around, and wag his tail in excitement when I come home. Jonathan Balcombe (2006), an animal behaviourist, shows that dogs and other animals share our capacities for empathy, humour, and aesthetic pleasure. Moreover, contra Aristotle's understanding of human-to-human relationships, my human to animal relationship is unlikely to dissipate and break off, for it is extremely satisfying and valued by Harry and me, in addition to which the circumstances of our relationship are unlikely to change significantly in the foreseeable future.

A friendship of utility is one in which the parties provide mutual advantages for one another. The friendliness that depicts this sort of relationship is largely based on the usefulness that is served by being pleasant to one another, for example, in a workplace. Again, says Aristotle, there is little to sustain the relationship when the mutual utility ends. In my relationship with Harry, there is a kind of mutual usefulness operative. Through Harry, I satisfy certain psychological needs, for example, for affection, loyalty, and comforting tactile contact from a dependent being, while he benefits from me in that his physical and psychological needs for food, shelter, stimulation, and affection are regularly satisfied. As this mutual pleasure giving is central to our relationship, contra Aristotle, it is unlikely to end, barring exceptionally bad circumstances.

Finally, there is the friendship of excellence or character. Such a friendship is mainly characterized by two "virtuous" people wishing the best for one another. (For Aristotle, virtue refers to some human excellence, intellectual or moral. To have moral virtue, for example, is to have developed one's character in such a way that one habitually chooses the mean between the extremes of excess and deficiency.) While such relationships are, of course, pleasurable and useful, such aspects are secondary, because these people wish the best for their friends mainly for their friends' own sake. According to Aristotle, such friendships emanate from good character, and, thus, the individuals involved must be virtuous already, or rather one of them must be virtuous while the other one is characterized by the likely possibility for developing virtue, something the first person will assist in developing. Such relationships are not common, because they require substantial time and effort to develop and nurture.

While Harry has his functional importance to me, the fact is that I also wish him well for his own sake. Harry is a fellow living creature, one that does no harm to other living beings, is one of God's creations, a manifestation of the Tao, that mysterious force that determines all things and embraces all forms of being, and I want him to live a long and happy life, to be the best dog he can be, according to his own nature, in his own way and time. Moreover, I experience Harry as "wanting" the same for me through his joy-inducing non-verbal modes of communication and life-affirming felt presence. In other words, in some sense, both Harry and I participate in the vital rhythms of Nature, and this involves a degree of wishing the other well, that is, in working together in giving joyful form to our lives together. For me, this is in part a matter of apprehending the interlocking and interdependent relationships between the multiplicity of parts of the universe, in this case my relationship with Harry, and to derive a feeling of connectedness and contentment at viewing myself as organically related to his world and as belonging to the universe as a whole. For Harry, as Freud insinuated about Jo-fi, such "simplicity of a life, free from the almost unbearable conflict of civilization . . . the beauty of an existence complete in itself" instinctively manifests, or at least implies, a similar Nature-animated wisdom. Harry "wants" me to flourish, as I do him, because we are both constituent elements of the same web of interconnectedness and interdependence in the universe, a living, organic universe animated by Nature or, in religious language, by God. In this sense, there is a sacred bond that unites "The Pup" and me.

There have been a few especially noteworthy instances, however, when Harry's concern for my well-being, more or less for my sake, seemed to be strikingly manifest. I am thinking about the time I had an allergic reaction to some wheat I accidentally ate which lead to an anaphylactic reaction, causing me almost to pass out before I could get to my Epi-pen adrenalin injector. In this moment of panic and horror, I was in the kitchen while my wife was in her office, unable to hear my cries for help. As I lay on the floor, losing consciousness, Harry began to bark furiously, in a manner that was entirely out of character as he is not, in general, a barker, causing my wife to interrupt her session and come to see what was wrong. Indeed, if Harry did not make his atypical barking and commotion, my wife would not have left her session and I would not have been able to get the injection I needed. Clearly, Harry was troubled that something was wrong, or at least unnerving to him, and if he had not sounded the alarm I might have died. It is, of course, easy and tempting to assign human motivation to an animal, including altruistic-like motivation, but such an experience as I had, and there are thousands of similar stories of dogs saving their masters, does make one wonder if there is more going on in a dog's mind and heart than simply the anthropomorphic interpretations that we, as cynics claim, mistakenly assign to a dog's human-like, devotional behaviour. Indeed, humourist Josh Billings was probably right when he quipped that dogs are the only things on the planet that love you more than you love yourself (Balcombe, 2006, p. 156).

Harry as a love object: "affection without ambivalence"

One cannot help but remember Picasso's devoted friend and beloved dog, Lump, who was the painter's inseparable companion during the later years of his life and the subject of a series of masterpieces in the Picasso Museum in Barcelona (*AARP Magazine*, 2006, p. 20). Similarly, Mozart rewrote a section from the last movement of his Piano Concerto in G Major to match the beautiful song of his beloved pet starling (Balcombe, 2006, p. 176), and to understand better why Freud believed that we can "love an animal with such extraordinary intensity . . . affection without ambivalence" it is necessary to briefly explore Freud's views on the psychology of love.

For Freud, all love relations are a "refinding of the object", roughly analogous to the emotional experience of symbiotic togetherness with the mother or care-giver. What this means in terms of establishing love relations is that, to some extent, the choice of our significant other repeats or calls to mind aspects of our childhood care-givers. Love, says Freud, "consists of new editions of old traits and it repeats infantile reactions" (Freud, 1915a, p. 168). That is, all love is based on infantile templates and is fundamentally a fixation on the parents, what Freud calls transference love. According to Fine (1979, p. 48), transference love and ordinary love differ only in terms of degree. The problem with this, of course, is that if we refind that which is "bad" from our childhood experiences, it usually leads to impoverished and/or destructive intimate relationships. The trick, then, is to refind in the significant other that which is consciously and unconsciously "good" from our childhood care-givers, so that we and our partners have a better chance of being happy in our love relation.

For Freud, however, to accomplish this seemingly straightforward task is not at all simple, for it requires resolving at a higher level of personality integration at least three aspects of love: "narcissistic versus object love; infantile versus mature love; hate versus love" (Moore & Fine, 1990, p. 113). To the extent that love is dominated by inordinate, unhealthy, and pathological narcissism (e.g., self-centredness and selfishness), infantile and dependent wishes and behaviour (e.g., the other exists mainly to gratify one's needs and wishes on demand), and hate (e.g., heightened ambivalence), one's love relation is doomed to failure. To the extent that it is animated by altruistic concerns (e.g., enhancing the other), is mature (e.g., recognizes that the separate other has needs and wishes worthy of gratifying), and is mainly affectionate (e.g., not corrupted by aggression), it is likely to succeed. For Freud, and this needs to be emphasized, all relationships are ambivalent. However, ultimately, the precondition to maintaining a stable, healthy, mature love relation is that affectionate sentiments towards one's significant other are much stronger and pervasive than the aggressive ones.

For Freud, as is well known, love is to be understood within a closed energic paradigm and instinctual outlook, all forms of love being derivatives of instinct with the function of giving instinctual gratification. For Freud, all love is love of a need-satisfying object. Mature object love, in contrast to infantile, dependent, need-satisfying love, is love that recognizes the reality of the other, that is, his otherness, his being a separate person with needs and wishes requiring and deserving gratification. Perhaps most importantly for Freud, the capacity for mature love requires object constancy, the capability to maintain an enduring relationship with a specific, single, separate other. This, in turn, presupposes the development of both a stable, structurally sound, coherent self and secure internalized object relations. Normal love, says Freud, thus results from the blending of caring, affectionate, and sexual feelings towards a person of the opposite sex (now we would say "significant other"). Its accomplishment is characterized by genital primacy in sexuality and by object love in relationships with others.

Freud saw love relations, actually all human relations, as largely reflecting a utilitarian motive, that is, of using the other to gratify biologically endowed drives and, thus, as a means to one's end. As Kleinian analyst Donald Meltzer points out (Meltzer, 1978, p. 84, cited by Alford, 1998, p. 128), for Freud, loving is like opening up a factory, of making a kind of capital investment bent on generating a profit. One does not invest libido unless one feels fairly sure that one will get back more than one gives. For Klein, on the other hand, love is conceptualized more in terms of bequeathing to a charity. As Alford further says (*ibid.*), "love gets from the very act of giving. It gets the opportunity to repair the self by repairing and restoring the world, or at least a little part of it". For Melanie Klein, love emanates from the infant's sense of gratitude towards the "good" mother; in Kleinian language, towards the satisfying, "good breast". This feeling is the basis for the infant's and later the adult's "appreciation of all goodness in the self and others" (Bergman, 1987, p. 248).

What on earth does my relationship with Harry have to do with all of this abstract Freudian love theory?

First, as Freud indicated, all human love relations are "refinding of the object", that is, they are "new editions of old traits and it [a love relation] repeats infantile reactions". In my case, Harry probably represents the gratification of selfobject needs that I never had adequately satisfied as a child by my depressed father and narcissistic mother. A selfobject is someone, in this case Harry, who strengthens and sustains the sense of self, that is, the self's cohesion, firmness, and harmony. As I have suggested, Harry is never boring, hackneyed, or graceless; rather, he is vibrant, alive, and always a surprise to my soul. Harry as an enlivening, invigorating and surprising Other was demonstrated quite clearly to me when I suddenly decided to bring him to a psychotherapy session with a wayward, extremely resistant, court-mandated adolescent who had not spoken to me, or hardly acknowledged that I was in the office, for nearly six months. When Harry came dashing into my office, tail wagging and bouncing about, and then started delightfully to engage the young man, almost miraculously the young man's hermetically sealed character armour gave way to a humanity and relatedness, first to Harry, and then to me, that was striking. Our discussion about my "dog friend", as I referred to Harry, evoked a desire in the young man to tell me about his dog that, incidentally and luckily, apparently looked similar to Harry. This episode proved to be most important as it became the young man's way, and my way, to engage each other in meaningful and emotionally important dialogue. Thus, thanks to Harry, the treatment was off and running. Harry remained in my office for all subsequent sessions, at times even lying underneath the young man's chair while he gently stroked his soft fur.

Harry evokes a kind of enhanced sense of integration that was, in many ways, lacking in my early development as a consequence of inadequate parenting. What has been refound, as it were, through a corrected version, is the opportunity to be the "good enough" care-giver that, at the same time, makes me feel more enlivened, significant, and whole. I experience Harry as a living being that gives me a sense of comfort, healing, and happiness through our giving and receiving love, each in our discernible respective human and animal ways.

As I have indicated, for Freud, to the extent that the love is characterized by self-centredness and selfishness, the significant other is viewed as existing largely to gratify one's needs and wishes on demand, and therefore entails heightened ambivalence, with one's love relations likely to fail. A so-called healthy love relation, in contrast, has at least three interrelated features that are, in general, operative: (1) it is other-directed and other-regarding, (2) it is "mature," that is, it is not infantile, dependent, and needy, (3) it is affectionate. Such is my relationship with Harry.

Thus, (1) I have a strong wish to enhance Harry, to keep him healthy and happy, mainly for his sake, though I, too, benefit from his flourishing in his life-affirming "dogness"; (2) I also recognize that Harry is a separate other, one that has needs and wishes worthy of gratification that at times have almost nothing to do with my self-serving needs and desires. As happens in the infrastructure of any close relationship, I make an effort to take Harry's needs and wishes into consideration as I interact with him, trying to synchronize our togetherness to be mutually satisfying. Sometimes his needs come before mine, as when I want to go to sleep rather than take him for a late night pee, or I stop what I am doing to pet him when he seems to be asking for it; (3) finally, my relationship with Harry is not marred by aggression or hostility; in fact, as Freud himself experienced, unlike human relationships, my relationship with Harry is characterized by a lack of marked ambivalence, that is, it is almost always warm, friendly, and affectionate. Indeed, as my mother-in-law once correctly noted, she did not recall my being as consistently pleasant and cheerful to my two children when they were infants.

While these observations, largely based on Freud's speculations on the secret of his love relation with Jo-fi, or at least my rendering of it, are illuminating, there is something missing in Freud's account. There is more to this relationship than is embodied in Freud's insightful, naturalistic, biological, pleasure/utilitarian animated remarks to account for what makes Harry so irresistibly appealing, if not loveable. Following Levinas, I suggest that what has been neglected, obfuscated, or overlooked by Freud and others is the realm of responsibility, purpose, and meaning that is the foundation of my love relation with Harry: call it "The Pup's" summoning, commanding "ethical address" (Atterton, 2004, p. 270). I believe that Harry, or any beloved dog for that matter, has a profound ethical significance. It is an ethical exigency that appeals to the goodness, kindness, generosity, and selflessness of what Levinas describes as the responsible self. In a word, it is the evoked suffering in me for Harry's real and symbolic suffering, in the same, or at least a similar way as with fellow humans, that constitutes Harry as ethical address (*ibid.*, pp. 270–271).

Harry as ethical address

Recall my first encounter with Harry in his Queens foster home. I described him as "very skinny and fearful, with long floppy ears and sad eyes". Moreover, I noted that he was a "rescue" dog who had been "abused and abandoned, a stray found on the highway, starving, filthy with fleas and tics and very frightened". Finally, and perhaps most importantly, both my wife and I felt a spontaneous summoning call from Harry: "Help me, love me, take good care of me."

By way of concluding this chapter, and towards provisionally answering Freud's question as to why a human can love his dog with such "extraordinary intensity", I want to unpack the above observations of my first encounter with Harry using Levinas's philosophy of the Other, his "ethics of responsibility" as my main hermeneutic resource.

Levinas has suggested that it is in the face-to-face encounter with another human, though he did make reference once to the face of a dog (Levinas, 1988, p. 169), that the other's alterity, his otherness, that which cannot be made intelligible by consciousness, is uniquely manifested and expressed. The face is Levinas's metaphor, says Wyschogrod (2000), for "the disincarnate presence of the Other", it is "the source of revelation of the other who cannot be encompassed in cognition" (p. 244). Thus, the Other can never simply be reduced to one of my ideas or conceptions. Perhaps most importantly, says Wyschogrod, the face "calls separated being, egoity, the self into question" (*ibid.*). That is, the face is radically disruptive and strangely and irresistibly morally summoning and obligating. When one actually encounters the face of the Other, and even more importantly in terms of the face's ethical significance, the face assigns me to my self, in responsibility, without necessarily being able to imagine, conjure up, or thematize the other for whom I am responsible. Moreover, the face does not signify the Other in the manner that a sign does when it presents a meaning to an observer who can take hold of it and reduce it to objectified, comprehensible significance. Rather, says Levinas, the face as enigmatic alterity signifies an irreducible order or command to respond to the Other, but signifies it as being prior to my being psychologically present to respond. It is a kind of non-conscious moral desire, a primordial stirring in one's soul, to use religious language. Moreover, once affected by the Other, by his vulnerability, weakness, and suffering, the responsible self is "hostage" to the Other. He feels morally obligated and responsible to tend caringly to the Other's needs and wishes, to enhance the Other's life with the fullness of his whole being. Says Levinas, "the word 'I' means to be answerable for everything and for everyone" (Levinas, 1996a,

p. 90). Moreover, this responsibility for the Other is asymmetrical and non-reciprocal; it is not based on the common assumption of most adult relationships in our culture, "I am for you, you are for me." Such responsibility is "for the Other", not "for oneself".

Thus, conceived as the vulnerable, weak, suffering Other, and as a dog, Harry is more other than any human Other; he evoked a call that affected me before I was psychologically present to conceptualize it. This summoning call, this epiphany of the face, as insinuated from Harry's pained and destitute countenance, moved me, as do "the widow, the orphan, the poor, the stranger", the Others that Levinas has in mind. As Atterton points out, one thinks of Nietzsche, who, seeing a horse being beaten cruelly and pitilessly by a coachman, threw his arms around the horse's neck and collapsed, irreversibly insane. Atterton continues, "His final breakdown—and break with the world of humans—was brought on by the sight of a horse being tormented. He suffered for the unjustifiable suffering of a horse" (Atterton, 2004, p. 279). Like these vulnerable and defenceless human Others, Harry commands an ethical response, one like that of the biblical Abraham, who heard the commanding call from God and responded, "Here I am!" It is through this responsibility for the Other, human- and, I believe, animal-directed, that one's capacity to love emerges in full splendour, for it is love as a sacrifice of self, a gratuitous devotion to the Other, before oneself. This is precisely what Levinas means by the ethical relation.

What I am suggesting is that through my relationship with Harry, I realize my ethical obligation to be responsible to and for the Other. While this notion is largely understood by Levinas in terms of the human-to-human encounter, the same, or at least similar ethical call can apply to a human-to-animal relationship, in this case, to be open and accessible, and to assist Harry. Harry, in other words, has ethical exigency that demands an ethical response. As Morgan has further noted (2005, pp. 7, 9, 11), Levinas made it clear that only in situations of genuine difference and otherness (and what is more Other to a human than a dog?), where one acts on behalf of the Other, can ethics be said to actually be present. Harry teaches me, even "trains" me, to hear the demand, the cry of the Other, to be receptive and responsive to the radically Other, and this means, in many instances, suppressing my narcissism and selfishness to put his needs before mine as any good dog owner routinely does.

Through mindfulness of Harry's vulnerability, as with one's infant child, a living being utterly dependent on me for his survival and happiness, I become aware of the ineluctability of my ethical responsibilities. Harry is thus a kind of "training ground" for acting on my obligations towards humans, especially those who are marked by extreme otherness (*ibid.*, p. 9). I am here thinking of the vulnerable, weak, and hated others of our world. That one chooses to take on the responsibilities of taking care of a dog emphasizes the fact that human subjectivity is "knotted in ethics" conceived as responsibility for the Other. The human face, and, I believe, the animal's face, orders and ordains me, says Levinas, as when one says, "Someone's asking for you." It is a demand that signifies a call to "giving and serving" the Other (Levinas, 1985, pp. 95, 98, 119).

Why, then, do we "love an animal . . . with such extraordinary intensity; affection without ambivalence", as Freud claimed?

My answer to the above question speaks to a striking paradox: that it is through one's relationship with a vulnerable, needy, defenceless animal, one that is radically other, that one becomes fully human, a giving and serving self in which love, conceived as responsibility for the Other before oneself is the primary affect-integrating, meaning-making, and action-guiding basis of the relation. Indeed, as I have suggested, that while I clearly derive instrumental satisfaction from my relation with Harry, what makes my relationship with him uniquely satisfying, in some sense analogous to raising a loved infant, is that it provides me with a context for loving in a way where the ethical aspect overrides the passionate one. It is through the day-to day taking good care of my hound, amid the dehumanizing pressures of my busy, if not frantic, life, that I reclaim my human dignity. As Hassidic Rabbi Shlomo of Karlin said, "The greatest sin a Jew [i.e., a person] can commit is to forget that he is a prince" [that he has a divine aspect to his soul].

In light of this last point, as with the story of Freud and his beloved Jo-fi that began this essay, I want to end by mentioning a poignant anecdote that Levinas tells about "Bobby", a dog that he came to know while interned in a Nazi-administered prisoner of war camp as a French officer from 1940–1945. In this camp, where Levinas did forced labour in the forest, the Jewish prisoners were separated from the others and forced to wear a patch with the word "*JUD*" on their clothing, and suffered other indignities and hardships. Once, says Levinas, when he was marched to and from his work through the French streets under the hateful, anti-Semitic stares of the onlookers, it was Bobby (as the prisoners named him), who would appear at morning assembly and was waiting for them as they returned, jumping up and down and barking in delight. Says Levinas, while the onlookers "stripped us of our human skin . . . [and we felt] no longer part of the world . . . for him [Bobby], there was no doubt that we were men" (Levinas, 1990a, pp. 151–153). For Levinas, it was this dog, not the human onlookers, who attested to the dignity of the prisoners.

Levinas's moving description of Bobby calls to mind the other Bobby of legendary fame, a Sky Terrier who was the close companion of John Gray, who died in 1858.

> Though dogs were not at that time officially permitted in the cemetery where Gray was buried, Bobby refused to be discouraged by the cemetery keeper's attempts to keep him out. On the third day after Gray's burial, as Bobby lay at the mound of earth during a cold rain, the keeper took pity and brought him some food. Thereafter, Bobby had free access to the cemetery, and for the next fourteen years the dog never spent a night away from his master's tomb. [Balcombe, 2006, p. 147]

There are a statue and fountain honouring Bobby's love and devotion that was erected in 1873. His headstone reads, "Let his loyalty and devotion be a lesson to us all" (*ibid.*).

Bobby, Jo-fi, and my Harry, through their "friendly growling" and "animal faith" (Levinas, 1990a, p. 153), through their unassuming sweetness and goodness, signify what can only be called transcendence. It is the transcendence manifested, expressed, and renewed through an elemental, though hugely summoning, ethical relation, one that calls to mind an impossible-to-satisfy debt, except perhaps, and only partly, through an abiding gratitude to "man's best friend".

CHAPTER TWO

Victory through vegetables: self-mastery through a vegetarian way of life*

> "The odd thing about being a vegetarian is not that the things that happen to other people don't happen to me—they all do—but they happen differently: pain is different, pleasure different, fever different, cold different, and even love different"
>
> George Bernard Shaw

While Shaw was being humorous in his letter to Ellen Terry, he was also making an observation that rings true to this psychoanalyst. For some time now, having treated a few analysands who were vegetarians, I have been wondering to myself what makes such people tick, those who live a "vegetarian way of life". By a vegetarian way of life, I mean those individuals, like Pythagoras, Tolstoy, Shelley, Einstein, and Leonardo Da Vinci, to name a few famous vegetarians, who have, to varying degrees, an almost visceral contempt for what they view as the unnecessary killing of animals, who are greatly concerned about animal welfare, earth ecology, and maintaining good physical

*An earlier version of this essay appeared in the *Psychoanalytic Review* (2008).

health. Such lacto-vegetarians (see below) are often associated with progressive social thought, though there have been a few infamous exceptions like Adolph Hitler and Richard Wagner (an unrepentant anti-Semite).

As Fox points out (1999, p. 55), vegetarianism is an umbrella term for a wide range of types: lacto-vegetarians eat dairy products, but no eggs or meat (about 70% of the world vegetarians are lacto-vegetarians); lacto-ovo vegetarians consume eggs and dairy products, but not meat; ovo-vegetarians eat eggs, but do not eat dairy products and meat; vegans do not eat meat, dairy products, or eggs (and often no honey as well); macrobiotic vegetarians consume only whole grains, sea and land vegetables, nuts and beans. There are also natural hygienists, raw foodists, semi-vegetarians and non-interventionist vegetarians. Vegans regard themselves as the "high priests" of the vegetarian community, the only true and properly consistent vegetarians, though that is hotly disputed by other vegetarians. Like religion, or for that matter psychoanalysis, vegetarianism can be life-affirming or life-denying, depending on the individual who embraces such a social practice. More generally, understanding the vegetarian way of life, which, of course, includes a vegetarian "state of mind", raises profound matters that are relevant to more general psychological issues of interest to psychoanalysis: what people eat, their diet, is an important statement and symbol of what they believe and feel strongly about, mainly because food consumption is an everyday activity, one that is crucial for their survival, their sense of well-being, and their social identity (e.g., think of the all of the ritual and ceremony associated with eating) (Spencer, 2000, p. x). If the food one eats is an important component of the social construction of self-identity ("you are what you eat") (Fox, 1999, p. 25), this means that eating has many conscious and unconscious meanings that are relevant to understanding a particular analysand's way of being in the world (Spencer, 2000, p. x). This is especially the case when we consider why people choose to give up eating meat (as opposed to those raised in a vegetarian culture like Gandhi), where eating meat is generally regarded as a common pleasure of omnivorous humans, at least in Western culture. Moreover, the psychology of meat-abstention is particularly interesting in light of the fact that abstainers have to endure the mockery and even anger of meat-eaters, a common response from non-vegetarians in our culture. While much more accepted in popular culture than in earlier times, vegetarianism is still often regarded as a culturally disruptive, if not subversive, activity.

Most importantly, and this is the main question I wish to address in this chapter: how can embracing a vegetarian way of life contribute to the development of greater autonomy, integration, and self-mastery? More specifically, I will argue that the ethical values that are lodged in the vegetarian way of life, such as non-violence (e.g., rejecting unnecessary animal suffering and death), unreasonable exploitation of Nature (e.g., environmental spoilage), the respectful acceptance and affirmation of the Other (e.g., inter-species kinship), and planet survival (e.g., world hunger) are ultimately animated by what analysts would call "mature" ethical emotions of love and compassion (Fox, 1999, p. 61). Such life-affirming valuative attachments, characterized by relatedness and gratitude, in contrast to an entitlement attitude of "proprietorship, instrumentalism and domination" (*ibid.*, pp. 60–61, 101) are in harmony with the ethical values and the celebration of life that constitute the psychoanalytic outlook at its best. Indeed, as Freud wrote to Jung, psychoanalysis is "a cure by love" (McGuire, 1974, pp. 12–13), and it is this alliance with Eros, as opposed to Thanatos, that constitutes the vegetarian way of life at its best. As one vegetarian pithily told me, "I want my body to be a monument to the living rather than a graveyard for the dead."

In an attempt to answer this question, how can embracing a vegetarian way of life enhance one's self-mastery and ethical subjectivity, I will present excerpts from an analysis of a young man who decided to become a lacto-vegetarian while in treatment. I will also use data from a number of interviews with acquaintances of mine who are vegetarians. For the record, I, aged fifty-six, have myself been a lacto-vegetarian for most of my adult life.

The world of the vegetarian

Like motorcyclists, baseball devotees, and stamp collectors, the vegetarian is part of a community of like-minded people who have deeply felt, shared values and quasi-ritualized activities. By way of contextualizing my case vignette and the discussion that follows, I therefore want to make some observations about the "typical" vegetarian, his relationship to the natural world, the trajectory leading to his giving up eating meat, and his new community. Roughly 1–2.8% of adults in the USA are vegetarians, too large a number to make any meaningful generalizations about. Therefore, I will limit my brief, speculative comments to those individuals who chose to be vegetarians in adolescence or adulthood, and who live in western societies. Such were the vegetarians I interviewed, as was the analysand I will describe in the case vignette.

There are many reasons why a person chooses to become a vegetarian, or at least there are many thoughtful philosophical / religious arguments for doing so, arguments that I will not review. Whatever the conscious moral reasons for giving up meat-eating (perhaps excluding those who do so only for health concerns), vegetarians usually have somewhere in their stated outlook the notion that they see themselves as "*part* of Nature, rather than *apart* from Nature" (Fox, 1999, p. 176, original italics). In their minds, choosing vegetarianism is an attempt to reconfigure "the human–animal relationship" on a more "harmonious" basis, where cruelty, brutality, and exploitation no longer dominate. In other words, Fox continues, most vegetarians have decided that the best way of fitting within and relating to the natural world is to embrace "compassionate cohabitation". Such ethically-infused, affect-animated desires for "connection and relatedness, reciprocity and community" are, thus, some of the regulative values for what vegetarians regard as living the reasonable, moral "good life" (*ibid.*, pp. 110, 176).

Often, what first brings a person to consider the possibility of giving up eating meat is some kind of intense emotional identification with the suffering animal world. In vegetarian circles, such identificatory moments have been called "meat insight experiences" (Amato & Patridge, 1989, p. vii). That is, while eating meat, the person is overwhelmed with troubling fantasies and images of living animals, perhaps even of pets, or cut up animals on display at the butcher or in the supermarket, that lead him to feel intense moral revulsion. One vegetarian I interviewed indicated that he could not finish eating his pork chop when he noticed the dead, roasting pig on a rotating skillet in his favourite Greek restaurant. Another interviewee told me that when she was tearing the meat off a scrumptious turkey leg on Thanksgiving Day, she began to imagine it was the leg of her beloved cat. Sometimes these meat-eating insights are extreme, if not grotesque: "I first seriously decided to do without meat when my mother cooked my pet rabbit in a stew and I ate it without knowing it. [Needless to say, he found out soon after.]" (Fox, 1999, p. 56).

While such reactions are psychoanalytically complex, what is most striking about these reactions is that the usual defences that people have in our culture that allow them to separate their favourable feelings about the meat they eat from the feelings they have for other animals, pets, for example, break down, causing an impossible-to-ignore psychological condition. In other words, the vegetarian is not able to maintain the splitting of thought and feeling that allows him to think that the beautifully garnished cow, sheep, pig, chicken, or fish on his dinner plate is a creature that has suffered terribly, in, for example, factory farming, but is somehow not a member of the same group of living, sentient beings as our beloved dog, cat, rabbit, bird, or goldfish. As one teenage female vegetarian recently told me, "I became a vegetarian when I realized that the cow I was eating was a mammal with feelings just like me."

As I have insinuated, the vegetarian community is made up of a wide range of individuals who somehow share certain moral, social and political commitments based on the core conviction that eating meat is morally wrong, that it reflects a selfish, ultra-anthropocentric, misguided attitude towards the sentient world. Meat-eaters unashamedly assert that humans have the right to kill the "Other", that is, sentient life that is perceived as radically different and alien. For the vegetarian, the killing of conscious, mindful, and feeling creatures is experienced as radically unacceptable and guilt-inducing, if not sinful. Such socially sanctioned killing does not reflect an attitude of what Levinas famously calls "responsibility for the Other", the caring and respectful attitude towards the Other, before oneself, that constitutes what Levinas, and, for that matter, most great world religions and spiritual traditions (Marcus, 2003) regard as the ideal self–other, self–world relation. The question that immediately comes to mind for the psychoanalyst is, why does the vegetarian choose to so intimately link his eating habits to his moral commitments, that is, to eat in a way that is not dedicated to his own pleasure-seeking, but rather, to the well-being of animals, fellow humans, and the planet? It is to this important question that we now turn.

Freud's study of Leonardo Da Vinci

Freud had a long-standing interest in Leonardo in terms of the psychology of the artist. His study (1910c) was the first, and his only, full-length psychoanalytic biography ever written, one that provides the reader with a model for applying the insights from clinical psychoanalysis to an important historical figure. Freud's study has two parts: first, an investigation of Leonardo's personality and its connection to his creative work and achievements, and second, the search for the infantile basis of this remarkable contribution in Leonardo's actual childhood experience. Freud mentions in passing that Leonardo was a vegetarian as part of his summary of what he describes as Leonardo's generally kind and caring character. However, as Spencer notes and documents (2000, p. 178), Freud seemed to downplay the reality that Leonardo, one of the great humanists, actually had a fair amount of disgust for man himself, as did Freud. However, unlike Freud, Leonardo was a committed vegetarian. Wrote a lamenting Leonardo, "We make our life by the death of others" (*ibid.*, p. 179). This being said, I will quote three passages from Freud, to sensitize the reader to some of the important thematics pertinent to Leonardo that may also characterize the vegetarian way of being in the world.

> Leonardo was notable for his quiet peaceableness and his avoidance of all antagonism and controversy. He was gentle and kindly to everyone: he declined, it is said, to eat meat, since he did not think it justifiable to deprive animals of their lives; and he took particular pleasure in buying birds in the market and setting them free. He condemned war and bloodshed and described man as not so much the king of the animal world but rather the worst of the wild beasts. [Freud 1910c, p. 69]

Sounding like Leonardo, Freud wrote elsewhere, "I prefer the company of animals more than the company of humans. Certainly, a wild animal is cruel. But to be merciless is the privilege of civilized humans" (http://www.bearsmart.com/resources/quotes).

However, Freud also noted what can be psychoanalytically described as Leonardo's sadistic side, though wonderfully sublimated:

> But this feminine delicacy of feeling did not deter him from accompanying condemned criminals on their way to execution in order to study their features distorted by fear and to sketch them in his notebook. Nor did it stop him from devising the cruellest offensive weapons and from entering the service of Cesare Borgia as chief military engineer. [Freud, 1910c, p. 69]

Finally, concludes Freud,

> In an age which saw a struggle between sensuality without restraint and gloomy asceticism, Leonardo represented the cool repudiation of sexuality—a thing that would scarcely be expected of an artist and a portrayer of feminine beauty. [*ibid.*]

Thus, we have here three salient observations that are said to characterize Leonardo's inner life that may also characterize the "typical" vegetarian, if we can, for the sake of argument, reasonably assume such a category. Extrapolating from Freud, it is hypothesized that the typical vegetarian often presents to the outside world as gentle, kind, and progressive in outlook; he may have inordinate unconscious conflicts with his aggression, and he may be prone to self-denial in terms of sexual and other pleasures.

Kurt Eissler also wrote a psychoanalytic study of Leonardo (1962), in which he disagreed with such aspects of Freud's thesis as that Leonardo was on the edge of, if not barely fending off, depression. Eissler alleges that Leonardo had a "severe oral sadistic conflict" (*ibid.*, p. 60) and he therefore had to unconsciously fight off cannibalistic impulses when, for example, he was dissecting corpses. In Eissler's view, Leonardo's vegetarianism "permitted redemption of guilt by sacrifice and the sustenance of a potent defense . . . " (*ibid.*, p. 266). While both Freud's and Eissler's observations and formulations about the meaning of Leonardo's vegetarianism have been vigorously disputed by vegetarian-sympathetic social historians (Spencer, 2000, pp. 177–180), they impress me as good "food for thought" as we proceed in our psychoanalytic study, which is mainly aimed at suggesting how adopting vegetarianism can be part of an analysand's successful efforts at achieving a higher level of transformation of the self. Such a "new regime of the soul" (Hutter, 2006, p. 84), especially its enhanced other-regarding ethical expression, is what I mean by self-mastery.

Case vignette

Elie, age twenty-six, was a PhD student in literary studies when he first came to see me. He was having serious problems managing his doctoral adviser, who seemed bent on making his life hard going, perhaps to the point of hounding Elie out of the programme. Elie could not change his adviser, for his adviser was not only the only departmental expert in the subject Elie was researching, but also the longstanding, politically powerful head of the department. "He is my gatekeeper to getting my PhD," Elie told me. As a result of this precarious situation, Elie claimed that he was prone to depression, anxiety, and irrational fears of serious illness and premature death. He further indicated that he could not bear being so self-preoccupied, as was manifested in his more or less chronic anger and worrying, work addiction, and rumination about his lack of sexual/relationship fulfilment. Elie was not a vegetarian when I first met him. In fact, for reasons that will soon become clear, he tended to be a fast food consumer who also liked to snack on salty and sugary junk foods. Wise(r) potato chips was his favourite junk food (he used to eat nearly an entire large bag every night while watching television), while "medium rare" steak and baked potato smothered with sour cream was his favourite meal. Elie said that he "hated" vegetables, except for raw carrots (he liked their crunchiness).

Elie came from an upper middle-class Jewish family; his father was a well-known academic and his mother an accomplished editor. He had three older siblings who were also quite accomplished in their careers. Elie described his childhood as a difficult one, in that he had a domineering, critical, emotionally distant father, and a seductive and narcissistic mother, whom he nevertheless was strongly tied to. Elie was not a very good student from elementary school through high school, though he flowered once he went to college away from his parents. The most important aspect of Elie's history in terms of his turn to vegetarianism was his history of medical trauma as a child. At age four, he was hit by a car, sustaining a broken leg (he had playfully run away from his babysitter and into the street), and he was hospitalized for a few days. A few years later, at age eight, he required some additional surgery on his broken leg, though he never had any residual limp, only some episodic muscle and ankle pain. Elie came from a home where the idea of eating healthfully and staying fit was "pushed on me by my parents". There were very few snacks worth eating around the house, and his father, who had run a marathon a few times, was a jogging fanatic, while his mother, a very slim and good-looking woman, swam every day. Elie said that throughout his life his parents were irritatingly and excessively concerned about their health and fitness, and overbearing about maintaining his and his siblings' health, leading Elie to have his own stash of candy hidden in his bedroom and a disinterest in competitive sports (though he was naturally a good athlete, he claimed). As a result of his lack of exercise and poor eating habits, Elie was a bit overweight.

Elie turned to vegetarianism during what he called his "life and death" struggle with his PhD adviser, a rigid and demeaning man who seemed threatened by Elie, though Elie always impressed me as a rather nice young man, kind, thoughtful, funny, but also somewhat cynical and sarcastic. Elie says that he tried everything to please his adviser; however, no matter what he did, the adviser found a way to undermine, if not to discredit, his efforts. Elie said he did not know why the adviser took such a dislike to him, but he thought that the adviser may have been threatened by Elie's having come from such an intellectual Jewish background, in contrast to the adviser, who was a Baptist Southerner "from the aristocracy. His family probably had slaves," Elie was fond of saying. What was clear, said Elie, was that he was very angry with this adviser and felt largely powerless to engage him without the interaction turning to his disadvantage. Once, for example, when Elie was meeting with his adviser, his adviser mentioned an important book in their field that Elie should take a look at. Elie indicated that, by chance, he had read it a few months earlier. Said his adviser, "Well, well, Mr Literary Scholar from Long Island, maybe you should be the adviser and I should be the doctoral student." Elie, stunned by the adviser's defensive and nasty reaction, tried to explain respectfully what he meant, but the interaction became increasingly awkward and uncomfortable. Elie said that he often left his meetings with his adviser feeling humiliated and furious, and, later, depressed and anxious.

Elie said that he began to contemplate becoming a vegetarian when he happened by chance to discover in his university library a book about famous religious vegetarians. Reading those interesting reflections made him wonder about the ethical reasons for becoming vegetarian, so he began to research the subject. By that time he had given up eating junk food regularly, a diet that he viewed as a symbolic protest against his parent's hyper-healthy, controlling upbringing of him. He quietly began to change his meat-dominated diet somewhat, still eating meat, but less of it. When I asked him about this change in his eating habits, he told me that eating less meat and more vegetables (specifically mushrooms and avocado) was healthier and helped him keep his weight at his desirable level. Elie also said that he thought it was "sort of cool to be a veggie", though it was not exactly his thing; "Most veggies are weird," he cynically noted. It was within this context that Elie had his "meat eating insight" experience, actually two of them. In the first fantasy, while home for winter vacation and eating a chicken wing during dinner with his parents, he imagined he was devouring his childhood dog's paw. In the second fantasy, about a week later, while eating a piece of swordfish, he imagined he was eating his father's toes. After having both of these fantasies, Elie felt disgusted and could not finish his dinner. He also indicated to me that he must be psychotic to have such bizarre thoughts. The meaning of these cannibalistic fantasies was explored in his analysis.

As for the first fantasy, Elie indicated that his dog had always been his "best friend" in his difficult childhood, a source of comfort when he felt put upon by his demanding and critical father and rejected by his self-absorbed mother. He described going upstairs into his room and lying in his bed stroking his "doggie", as he called her. More importantly, Elie indicated that when he broke his leg and was hospitalized, he recalled fantasizing about his dog as a way of calming and amusing himself. In fact, Elie said that he had a very active and vivid fantasy life during his hospital stay and thereafter. He had a group of "animal friends", something akin to, though not exactly like, imaginary playmates who kept him busy at night and made him feel less alone and afraid. Elie said that neither one of his parents slept at the hospital, though they visited regularly. He did not recall many details of his hospital stay.

Elie believed that he had the fantasy of eating his dog's paw largely as a result of the heightened state of anxiety he was in concerning his adviser, further reinforced by being very angry with his father, who unfairly blamed him for not handling his adviser properly and jeopardizing his doctoral studies. Elie said that his father was very invested in Elie's following in his footsteps and getting a PhD in a related discipline. Elie hated this idea, but also recognized that he liked and was very good at literary studies, at least as long as he did not associate them with his father. The fantasy of ingesting his beloved dog's paw, Elie concluded, was thus a way of comforting himself while also expressing, in derivative form, his mainly oral sadistic wishes towards his hated father.

As for the second fantasy, imagining he was consuming his father's toes while eating a piece of swordfish, Elie indicated that he recalled that his father used to take off his socks and sneakers in the kitchen after jogging each morning and scratch his sweaty feet. His father's feet, he noted, had a colour similar to that of swordfish. Elie then made the connection between the word "sword" in swordfish and his wish to cut his father down to size. That is, Elie said that if he could have his way, his pompous and critical father would be psychologically "amputated" (hence eating his father's toes), as would his arrogant and nasty doctoral adviser, whom he associated with his father when he was most angry with him. "Both of these curly-haired idiots have ruled over me and made my life feel like shit," said Elie.

At the same time that these two fantasies occurred, Elie became considerably more anxious about his physical health, largely relating to two panic attacks he had while listening to a lecture (one given by his adviser), where he imagined that he was having a heart attack, forcing him to exit the lecture hall quickly and splash cold water on his face. Both panic attacks frightened him, as he had never in his life felt so scared for no obvious reason. "I felt completely out of control, trapped in a state of utter horror," Elie noted. Over time, Elie had become much more anxious about his overall health, both neurotically believing, and not believing, that he was suddenly going to die of a heart attack. Elie's anxiety got so bad that he sought out some anti-anxiety medication. The medication, combined with his understanding his panic attacks as largely a form of punishment for his rage-filled wishes against his adviser and, ultimately, his father, helped to reduce his fear of having another panic attack. Still, Elie's generalized anxiety was often uncomfortably high.

About a month later, Elie came into session and announced that he had decided to not eat meat any more, though he was going to continue to eat fish. He indicated that he felt that eating meat was "not a very nice thing to do to the poor cows". Fish, on the other hand, were more plentiful and did not suffer in factory farming, as did cows.

Having bought a number of books on the subject, Elie also became more and more interested in the philosophical and ethical bases of vegetarianism, finding the essays written by religious vegetarians the most interesting. Simultaneously, for a year or so, Elie became more religiously observant and interested in modern Hebrew literature. Both of these developments, giving up eating meat and becoming more observant, were understood by us as, in part, an attempt to modulate his angry and vengeful feelings towards his adviser/father, mainly by curbing his oral–sadistic impulses, while at the same time taking better care of himself by becoming involved in a nurturing religious community.

From the point of view of his developing vegetarianism, the next major moment was when Elie fell madly in love with a Jewish Studies doctoral student, an avid hiker, who was herself inclined towards vegetarianism. Though Elie had had a few important girlfriends over the years, he was always hesitant, tentative, and reticent about committing himself to a relationship. As far as I could tell, Elie had a tendency towards over-control and self-denial in his instinctual life. While he was functional in actual sexual relations, and a friendly and playful man, there was a defensive use of introspection, self-criticism, and thinking at the expense of the subrational, passionate side of him. As we shall see, the restrictions of a vegetarian diet allowed Elie to be freer in higher-level instinctual expression, as greater control over his oral–sadistic wishes allowed for greater progression into more age-appropriate and satisfying sexuality. Over time, as the relationship with this exciting, outdoors, and nurturing woman expanded and deepened, this "intellectually overloaded and top-heavy" man became a freer spirit (Hutter, 2006, p. 13). Indeed, Elie would describe hiking with his girlfriend in the mountains, engaging a Nature that was "largely unfiltered through social conventions", and that provided access to a dimension of being that he could neither fully understand nor describe, but which inspired him through its mysterious power and beauty (*ibid.*, pp. 69–70). Moreover, by feeling wonderfully nurtured by his girlfriend, Elie's early rage at his parents and his general neediness were greatly reduced, helping him to embrace life with less reserve. As part of this awakening to life and ensoulment, Elie and his girlfriend became lacto-vegetarians. They have become active on campus, promoting ecological awareness and enlightened social policy, including advocating vegetarianism. Incidentally, this case had a "happy ending". Elie married this woman. They are content with each other and plan to have children. He also completed his PhD, though not without increased hardship inflicted on him by his sadistic adviser. Said a proud Elie, "My face may be bloodied, but it is not bowed." Elie and his wife were now both looking for university teaching positions.

Vegetarianism as a form of "care of the self"

As this vignette suggests, vegetarianism can be used as a method for bringing about the transformation of a person's way of living, a "spiritual exercise", a way of working on oneself that supports human flourishing. For Elie, embracing a vegetarian way of life was understood as his effort at self-transfiguration through changing his "alimentary regime" (*ibid.*, p. 147). Such "experimental living", with its efforts at self-perfection and self-mastery, are best understood by what one Nietzsche scholar called the "care of the self", that is, self-cultivation of one's spirit, mind and body "in the service of something higher" (*ibid.*, pp. 125, 168).

What did Elie mean when he talked of "something higher"? How did he use a psychoanalytic technology of the self to achieve a higher form of integration? Finally, and most importantly for this chapter, how did Elie's embracing vegetarianism as a praxis of prudent living contribute to his psychic development and self-enhancement?

Elie was trying to transform himself from a self-described angry, pleasure-denying, self-punishing, and self-absorbed young man (his presenting agitated depression was highly narcissistic) into someone who could more freely give and receive love. An increased commitment and capacity to love, conceived as the "for the Other" responsibility, as Levinas describes it, was the valuative attachment that Elie regarded as his highest goal. Elie's turn to vegetarianism, while originating in infantile experience and neurotic conflict associated with his parents, managed to sublimate his anger, his narcissistic injury, into a more loving and compassionate outlook and way of relating to others. This shift in outlook and real-life behaviour was symbolized, expressed, and reinforced by his other-directed, other-regarding, life-affirming choice to abstain from meat on moral grounds, and in his increased capacity to love his girlfriend / wife. To the extent that Elie was able to use psychoanalysis to resolve, repair, and sublimate his various neurotic conflicts and self-deficits, rooted in his dysfunctional childhood, he was able to move to a "higher" level of ethical integration in which the rights of the Other, animal and human, took precedence over his infantile, selfish, and narcissistic needs and wishes. Elie's vegetarianism is, thus, best understood as a form of self-healing by means of a self-chosen ascetic programme, a diet characterized by self-sacrifice in the service of a joyful affirmation of life. In short, self-affirmation via self-denial, self-assertion in the service of self-creation. While Elie did not usually experience his vegetarian diet in any way as a deprivation, on some level he acknowledged it to be a form of instinctual renunciation that from time to time he felt unsettled about. This was especially the case as his character-based inhibitory, repressive, and excluding tendencies (*ibid.*, p. 71) were modulated through his analysis with the help of his earthy, pleasure-orientated girlfriend / wife.

It is also worth noting that, as Elie became more involved in his vegetarianism, not simply as a habituated alimentary regime (*ibid.*, p. 147) but as a way of life, he began to link it to a transcendental consciousness through his identification with the religious vegetarian traditions in Judaism and Hinduism, in particular. Though I felt that this turn in his thinking, which was related to his greater religiousness, was basically praiseworthy, I pointed out, and Elie agreed, that his capacity to embrace a new ascetic programme using religious sources represented his wish to legitimate his newly chosen way of life by using paternal authorities. It was also, in part, a way of further annoying his assimilated Jewish parents. Indeed, Elie was aware how irritated his parents were that he was a vegetarian, especially when his narcissistic mother, who took pride in her meat-based (though "lean cut"), French-style cooking, had to go out of her way to make sure that the food he ate was prepared properly and tasted good. Indeed, Elie's parents sometimes made snide comments about his unusual eating habits, as did some of his friends. Elie believed that their critical comments reflected their own guilt for eating meat, their sense of rejection by him of their lifestyle (especially his parents), and their envy of his greater self-discipline and ethicality. It did, however, also occur to me, and I put it to Elie, that at times he had a discernible, questionable sense of moral superiority and judgementalism because of his vegetarianism. Such a self-aggrandizing belief arrogantly asserts to meat-eaters: "I'm a better person than you". In addition, Elie had been somewhat of a maverick in his thinking and behaviour most of his life, and being a vegetarian satisfied this oppositional, if not subversive, side of him.

In closing this chapter, I want to point out that while vegetarianism may originate in neurotic conflicts and self-deficits, as in Elie's case, its meaning and function in adult life can be of such significance that it becomes a positive, psychologically healthy development. As with the adult opera singer I once analysed, who realized through her analysis that her choice of profession was partly rooted in her rage about not being listened to by her self-absorbed neglectful parents (her childhood shrill screaming she transformed into adult beautiful singing), so can a vegetarian's infantile, neurotic experience around food, health, and his overbearing parents be effectively sublimated. That being said, however, there are some vegetarians who chose to enact their vegetarianism for clearly and mainly neurotic reasons. Such people have some of the unresolved issues associated with patients who have eating disorders, extreme ascetic propensities, anhedonia, etc. Their vegetarianism can be viewed by the analyst as a sign of psychopathology. Though Elie never knew this, I was, as a vegetarian, in favour of his movement from an apolitical carnivore, junk food addict and couch-potato, to an environmentally active lacto-vegetarian, healthful eater, and devoted hiker. While I dutifully and vigorously analysed the neurotic aspects of Elie's choice to become a vegetarian and the collateral issues associated with his vegetarian way of life, I was also aware that his politics/ethics, in the broadest sense, and mine were in harmony, and this made our analytic work together that much more productive.

CHAPTER THREE

Long night's journey into day: on tending to a dying mother

> "I acknowledge the cold truth of her death for perhaps the first time. She is really gone, forever out of reach, and I have become my own judge"
>
> Sheila Ballantyne

"I want my momma, I want my momma," said a tearful Darell, aged nine, at our first psychotherapy session following the premature death of his mother from breast cancer. These pained words kept returning to my mind following the recent death of my eighty-nine-year-old mother from liver cancer. For Darell, in a simple, heartfelt, and poignant manner that perhaps only a child can express, conveyed what it felt like to be bereft of a mother, even to an adult son, one who is happily married with children, is established in his career as a psychoanalyst, and is settled in a comfortable lifestyle. Indeed, the death of a mother or, for that matter, a father or surrogate parent (though, in both cases, not exactly in the same way), often cuts deeply into one's being in an unprecedented and unpredictable manner. It radically disrupts that which one takes to be normal and normative, especially in terms of how one understands oneself and relates to others, particularly those one is close to. The sense of abandonment, the feeling of vulnerability, the idea of one's own mortality, the sense of the triviality, if not absurdity, of one's everyday life, are some of the well-known feelings associated with the loss of a loved one, especially of a parent, and even more so with the second parent who dies. In a word, one becomes inescapably aware that one is an "orphan," and this self-understanding is strangely, deeply troubling.

In this chapter, I want to suggest how a Levinasian-inspired, ethically-infused psychoanalytic outlook can, from two perspectives, significantly add to our psychological understanding of a parent dying, both from the perspective of the dying mother, and from the perspective of the adult son who helps tend to her. I will be focusing on how my elderly mother dealt with her approaching enfeeblement, illness, and death, and how this experience of witnessing her physical and mental deterioration and ultimate demise affected me. Thus, there is a double structure to this essay, parallel stories of her death and my life that intersect at the point of radical rupture of the world as she and I knew it. The first part of this essay is written within the sorrowful situation of a son who has lost his mother, while the second part is written more with the quasi-aloofness of the psychoanalyst. My hope is that these two forms of expression, testimonial and so-called detached analysis, mainly from a Levinasian perspective, will be illuminating, and possibly helpful, for others who have had to tend to an ageing and sick parent who is dying. Psychoanalysts, psychotherapists, and others working with such pained people may derive some new "food for thought" about this challenging and difficult life experience.

While there are extensive psychoanalytic, psychological, and literary studies on death and mourning (in the latter group, one cannot but think of Tolstoy's masterpiece, *The Death of Ivan Il'ich*, for example), some of it written from the perspective of an adult son or daughter dealing with a parent's death, my focus is on two aspects of this experience that have tended to be neglected, if not overlooked, in these literatures: first, the approach of death viewed as a modality of the relation with the Other, and, second, the approach of death as offering the possibility of perceiving a fundamental goodness that can be realized amid its violence and grief. As I will discuss later, a Levinasian perspective on the significance of death puts into sharp focus the realization that there is no more extreme encounter with alterity than in facing one's own death. Death is ambiguous, mysterious, and ultimately unknowable; it is also menacing. Being a "hostage" to death is thus a way of being a hostage to the Other. Levinas is here challenging Martin Heidegger's ontological outlook, his being-toward-death formulation in which death is viewed as the subject's ultimate trial of "mastery", "heroism", and "virility"—the possibilities of initiative (Levinas, 1987, p. 72). For Heidegger, the subject signifies the existential, that is, the uniqueness of subjectivity resides in facing death in anxious anticipation, revealing an authenticity that is judged by what is proper to me, what has already moved me (Kosky, 2001, pp. 125, 127). Instead, Levinas views death as unfathomable and radically disruptive, as pointing towards a mindfulness of otherness, of the face-to-face, in other words, of love as responsibility for the Other. In contrast to Heidegger's tragic–heroic paradigm, death thus signifies ethics, with the uniqueness of subjectivity residing in giving itself to the other, a pure gratuity towards, and sacrifice for, the Other. Heidegger and Levinas are, therefore, not so much talking about different types of subjectivity than they are pointing to two different orders in which subjectivity could possibly signify: the self as Being *vs.* the self as Goodness (*ibid.*). This interpretive difference is mainly rooted in their divergent views of the human condition, and on what they believe ultimately matters in life, including what constitutes being human at its best. Levinas scholar Richard Cohen aptly summarizes the matter, and underscores the second aspect of the significance of approaching death, including that of a parent, which I will later take up: its potential to be a source of goodness, especially for the survivors. Cohen writes that

> Levinas rejects Heidegger's analysis of being as being-toward-death, arguing that the death that matters most and cuts most deeply into my own psyche is not my own but the other's. Furthermore, it is not the other's death per se, but the other's mortality, meaning the other's aging and suffering, the other's vulnerability, that calls me to myself as responsibility for the other, responsible '"not to let him die alone". [Cohen, 2007]

In order to thoughtfully apply a Levinasian-inspired, ethically-infused psychoanalytic outlook to better understand the general psychological significance of the death of a mother, particularly the death of my mother, it is essential for me to tell you something about my mother so as to put her ageing, illness, suffering, and death into some kind of intelligible and meaningful psychological context. What better way to convey the essence of the woman, her life and death, at least as I viewed her, than to present the eulogy I gave at her funeral? This eulogy will, in part, serve as the "real-life" so-called "clinical material" for the rest of my essay, a kind of "case vignette" that I will often refer to and elaborate.

Eulogy for my mother

My mother's last wish was to have a eulogy with two characteristics: make it honest and make it short. I will honour the wish of this very complex and compelling woman, who, even as she faced death, and to her own detriment, never could be adequately comprehended or let herself be fully loved by those who cared about her. My mother was, and remains, something of a mystery to me, though my understanding of her became clearer towards the end of her life when she faced debilitating illness and death.

It is difficult to summarize a person's life in just a few minutes, even more so when the woman who died was eighty-nine years old. However, by way of giving you a sense of who my mother was, what she believed in, and how she lived her sometimes ennobling life, I will mention three key aspects of Sylvia Marcus, a daughter of immigrant parents, one of six children growing up in Washington Heights, New York, a graduate of New York University, a devoted wife of forty-plus years to my father. My mother did not have much to say that was positive about her upbringing; though her parents were dutiful, especially her mother, her father being remote, for the most part she felt disregarded and unsupported. These early experiences of lack of recognition and affirmation no doubt provided the basis for her stunning attempts to compensate for these early deficits, as my mother became one of the most commanding people I ever met, one of those people that it was impossible not to notice. Indeed, my mother knew how to grab your attention, engage you in fascinating dialogue, and make you feel that there was more to life than sham, drudgery, and broken dreams. Brutal honesty, especially about oneself, living through literature and teaching, and freedom of thought and imagination, were three major aspects of her life. I want to tell you a more about them.

Brutal honesty

If you want to know what a person thinks and feels deep down, find out two things: what quotes or pictures taken from a newspaper or a book they keep on their refrigerator or in a cupboard, and find out what they are most afraid of. Indeed, my mother's kitchen cupboard revealed what she valued and which people she most admired. There were quotes from Sartre, Camus, Kafka, Shakespeare, Golda Meir, Nelson Mandela, and Simone De Beauvoir. My mother felt that the only authentic way to engage life was honestly, not so much in terms of conventional ethics, though she was a decent person, but, more to the point, by facing who you are, without deception and fearlessly. I have memories from my childhood of my mother telling me and showing me, usually with a literary reference, that if you are going to be able to deal with the adversity of life, and if you are going to achieve a modicum of peace of mind, you had better "know yourself", the good and, especially, the bad aspects of your character. "I take life straight," my mother was fond of saying. What she did not know, of course, to quote one of my mother's favourite playwrights, Ibsen, was that if you "Take the saving lie from the average man . . . you take his happiness away, too". My mother had a depressive side to her, usually hidden, and it was never obvious when I was growing up, but, as she got older and became more cynical and isolated (her misguided choice to be a loner, for people always were drawn to her, and all of us frequently reached out to her), her personality became darker. Having lost her husband eighteen years ago, and having had a rough marriage for the last ten years of it, as she told us, as our dentist father had retired and was depressed himself, and having had to start a new life as a widower, my mother grew more pessimistic, though she fought her demons to the end, something very painful to watch.

Life as literature

Vladimir Nabokov, one of those authors who were represented in my mother's cupboard, wrote, "Literature and butterflies are the two sweetest passions known to man". My mother was unquestionably the best-read person I have ever known, at least with regard to world literature, and that includes my highfalutin' professor friends. My mother read all the books that we all should have read but never did. She knew the greatest European writers cold. Chekhov and the Russians were her favourites, and she often punctuated her conversation and storytelling—and my mother was one heck of a storyteller—with literary references and anecdotes. My mother read all of the Nobel Prize winners, and could masterfully critique them, and it was her life-long love of literature and her lecturing in various forums, at adult education classes, synagogues, and churches, museums, colleges, and on bus tours, that were when she was most in her element. Very smart, extremely psychological, disarming, incredibly engaging, and enormously entertaining was my mother lecturing and, for that matter, conversing at a dinner party—she always had her audience eating out of her hands in a few minutes and, as with a great movie, you did not want her to end. Hardly acknowledged as a child by her family, my mother had found a way of being heard and appreciated, of feeling significant, her most summoning need, in my view. Indeed, most people who spoke with her were quite willing to give her the space to talk, to do her thing; "lie back and enjoy the ride", I often felt. It was just that engaging and satisfying.

Freedom of thought and imagination

My mother raised me to think independently and to give my mind an opportunity to explore life wherever it took me. Ironically, and paradoxically, given her commitment to honesty, I also learned how important it was *not* to take life straight. As Cervantes wrote (and my mother thought highly of his work, though he never made it into her cupboard), "I imagine that everything is as I say it is, neither more or less, and I paint her in my imagination the way I want her to be". In other words, my mother figured out that, in a certain sense, we need our lies, we need to pretend, we need theatre in order to make life bearable, maybe even a bit pleasurable. My mother was an accomplished exaggerator and knew how to take the most mundane matter and make it into something special or unusual, sometimes even beautiful. Oscar Wilde, another favourite of my mom's, said that "Moderation is a fatal thing. . . . Nothing succeeds like excess". Of course, as my mother knew, the problem with such an approach to life was that when you have to face ordinary reality, it is often disappointing compared to the life of the imagination. But, as she told me, it was worth it, for, in her view, and this is the dark side of my mother, living was highly overrated.

There are other praiseworthy aspects of my mother that deserve mention. She was a kind woman, and a haven for some of you out there today, those of you who had "dead loss" parents who either gave up on you, were grossly inadequate, or just did not understand you. My mother gave encouragement and support to you, some of whom would probably have ended up living in a halfway house if it were not for my mother's emotional support; another fellow out there would have ended up in Creedmore Psychiatric Institute (Queens, New York). My mother was always kind to her extended family, generous in opening her home to others, and probably more forgiving than she should have been. My mother knew how to throw a great dinner party and Thanksgivings were always memorable. Her sense of humour was well-developed, though she could take an amusing swipe at anyone who got out of line.

My mother was very proud of her grandchildren, all of them, though she did not always reach out to them as much as she could have when she was with them; when she spoke about them, it was clear that she was connected and cared about them. She was also financially generous to them, as she was to her own children. However, it was probably as a mother-in-law that my mother was most unusual. This is because she didn't do the one thing that mothers-in-law frequently do, she didn't butt in and meddle. My mother knew her place, and that was to give her children's wives and husband the space they needed. She was always available to help when asked, though there were times when the distance she kept was experienced as disinterest and that hurt.

Likewise, as a mother she was kind and supportive, though, to be honest, and my mother wanted me to be honest in her eulogy, there were gaps in her parenting of my siblings and me. Not one of us can remember having had a birthday party as a child. At times, her remoteness, which increased as we got older, felt like rejection. Only later in life did we, now adults and ourselves parents, recognize and accept that my mother did the best she could given who she was and how inadequately she was raised. There are no perfect parents, but my mother was "good enough", as one famous psychoanalyst said. Indeed, my mother, who did almost all the parenting in our family, raised three good individuals, a bit neurotic perhaps, but it is a credit to her humanity and decency that my sister, Nancy, became a nursing instructor, my brother, Randy, a social worker, and I, a psychologist. Helping people, doing something that makes this misery-filled world a bit better, is mainly my mother living through us.

At the end of Sophocles' *Oedipus the King*, the chorus says, "call no man happy until you see how he has died". That is, getting the endgame wrong casts a shadow on one's whole life. My mother taught me something very deep and important about life, and this centrally included how to face death. You see, while my mother was dying, this fiercely autonomous and independent woman had to rely more and more on others to take care of her, and this, combined with the lessening of her physical powers, was extremely hard for her to deal with. This was a woman who walked three miles a day up until almost eighty-six and who called it "a great day" to be able to walk alone while communing with Nature, especially by the ocean, the place where she felt most at peace. My mother became angry and bitter as her liver cancer became more debilitating, and she seemed to put herself into a psychological cul-de-sac. For some reason, she had obliterated her past and was not able to sustain knowing and feeling that she had lived her life well, and, most important, that she had touched many people's lives in meaningful ways. In other words, my mother could not sustain herself as she lay dying through knowing that she would leave a lot of love behind. No, my mother felt it was all for naught, that she had not been a good person and was a selfish phoney. A harsh, unfair, and untrue verdict. In addition, by not being able to accept the love that she was given over the years, and there was a lot of it from her family and friends, she felt that her life and death were futile. In the end, having obliterated her past, and with no comforting transcendent world-view, sadly, my mother felt only nothingness, at times a terrifying nothingness, as she told me. This nothingness, her biggest fear, was equated with feeling utterly insignificant, probably similar to what she likely felt at her worst moments as a child. Interestingly, in one of her last coherent conversations with me, she acknowledged that her way of viewing her life, illness and death, was not "the right way", but she said that she could not help it. "Maybe it will change," she said. This was where her mind had taken her, rendering her trapped in a maze of grotesque happenings, with her literary imagination leaving her cold, depressingly withdrawing into herself. I felt at this point that I learned what *not* to do in terms of how to die, if one can actually determine such things. Though, as my mother told me, "No one really knows how you will deal with the end game when it is your turn." The fact is, as my mother's last autonomous act, before her capacities gave way, she willed herself into a more comfortable place, a kind of psychological oblivion. A coma.

"Don't mourn for me. Don't be sad," my mother told me in a more lucid moment towards the end. "I have had a good life for the most part." "Terrifying Nothingness" *vs.* "I have had a good life", two sides of a woman whose death and life will no doubt be a source of poignant reflection for me in the years to come. I have, despite her limitations, greatly benefited by my mother's efforts to help me become who I am. No serious regrets about my mom as a mother. I am grateful. I will miss her, terribly.

Death as an encounter with alterity

As the above eulogy insinuates, my mother's illness and approaching death was mainly experienced by her as a perilous confrontation with that which was like nothing she had experienced before, something menacingly, radically other, an inescapable horror that was impossible to articulate coherently. Put in more familiar psychological terms, her confrontation with her terminal illness and approaching death was perhaps somewhat analogous to what Bruno Bettelheim, a concentration camp inmate, called an "extreme" situation (Marcus, 1999). According to Bettelheim, when an individual is faced with an extremely confusing, rapidly changing, contingent reality, when routines and valued modes of thought and acting are in the process of being destroyed, one feels oneself to be in an "extreme" situation, in a social context in which one feels suddenly, massively, and decisively threatened with the destruction of his world. Such a situation almost always generates extreme conscious and/or unconscious death anxiety in one form or another. Indeed, my mother's illness, especially during the three months or so when she became increasingly aware that she was seriously ill and undeniably going to die, hurled her into a kind of "conceptual disarray", including the inability to put her disorganizing experience into a meaningful language, at least until she found a way of solving, as it were, the fundamental problem as she viewed it: how to leave this world with a modicum of autonomy and dignity.

Perhaps a useful way of further conceptualizing my mother's overall struggle with her ageing, illness, and approaching death, and, to a lesser extent, my struggle as her son witnessing her painful thrashing about and imminent death, is through the notions of "having a world, losing a world, and replacing a world" (Marcus, 1999, p. 73). By "having a world", I refer to what my mother had before her illness, to what Erving Goffman has called "a 'home world'—a way of life and round of activities taken for granted", until she became seriously ill (Goffman, 1961, p. 12). It was this home world that gave her, as it does all of us, a sense of direction in life and a feeling of safety and security. Once my mother became aware that she was terminally ill (especially after her doctor gave her approximately six months to live) and that she needed professional care-takers to help her with the most rudimentary routines, cooking, showering, toileting, and getting ready for bed, she gradually, with great resistance initially, had to face the fact that she had to give up her main ties to her home world. As she became sicker and more dependent on others for help, she more or less lost her entire social existence as she knew it before she became ill and was dying. To have such an awareness of the end of one's everyday life as one has always lived it, what I am calling "losing a world", is to be thrown into a relationship with that which is absolutely other. With the disappearance of my mother's familiar and security-generating pre-illness world, she became an "other" to herself. Her very personhood was transformed, as she had become irrevocably fractured and derailed and was no longer in possession of herself (Nemo, 1998, p. 43). Finally, as my mother went through the nightmarish experience of losing her world, with its regressive mode of self-experience—helplessness, humiliation, passivity, loss of individuality—she had to find or create a way of coping with all of this until she died. She had to generate a "replacement world", a way of thinking, feeling, and acting, a new inner centre of gravity, that would give a relative degree of order and direction to her life, that would make her suffering "sufferable", and imminent death tolerable, at least in some minimally self-comforting sense. This included her "new role", as she sarcastically described it, as the "dying mother"—a role that she vehemently hated, as she could not tolerate what she believed was others' pity, self-serving sentimentality, and looking to her as a kind of "oracle" who would spout great insights about life and death as she withered away. "I have no great insights," she told me, "I'm in an agitated abyss. I feel nothingness." Thus, bereft of her "home world", with her pre-illness world of meaning and sense of self more or less gone, she withdrew into herself. It is perhaps for this reason that, once my often cynical mother became undeniably sick, she never left her apartment except to walk a few steps in the usually empty hallway at unsociable hours, as her doctor had told her that this would help reduce the pain in her legs. Her apartment thus became the new context for her replacement world, a kind of protective cocoon that allowed her to fold ever more deeply into herself as she faced the suffocating tight circle of her illness.

Death, Levinas claims, is the ultimate encounter with alterity; it is an engagement with that which lies beyond Being, the Same, or the Ego (Davis, 1996, p. 30). That is, death is absolutely unknowable and, most evocatively perhaps, it is located in the dark realm from which murder comes.

> In death I am exposed to absolute violence, to murder in the night . . . the unwonted hour of its coming approaches as the hour of fate fixed by someone. Hostile and malevolent powers, more wily, more clever than I, absolutely other and only thereby hostile, retain its secret. [Levinas, 1969, p. 233]

What Levinas is getting at is that while my mother knew in some sense that when she would die was contingent, dependent on the future and in as yet unknown circumstances, she tended to think of the hour of her death as predestined by someone else. For Levinas, death, like a murderer, threatens from beyond, from the other, and "this alterity, precisely as absolute, strikes me in an evil design or in a judgment of justice" (*ibid.*, p. 234). Put more straightforwardly, my mother experienced her approaching death, at least at times, as if she was a hunted animal, as facing a predator who, for no reason that she could make adequate sense of, was out to get her and, even worse, despite her monumental efforts at escape (the "not yet" of death, there is still time), would ultimately find her, and kill her. Such a consciousness of hostility, of being in hand-to-hand combat with a superior and sadistic adversary, a kind of "pure menace", as Levinas describes it, is experienced as fear of sudden terrible violence. As author James Dickey famously described in his powerful novel *Deliverance* (1970), one of the greatest fears that humans have is to be suddenly set upon by an unexpected attack from a concealed position. The hour of death in some sense always feels like this, like an ambush.

What Levinas is noting, an insight that is not usually appreciated by those, including psychoanalysts, who are steeped in a Heideggerian analysis of death or its variations, is that "Death, in its absurdity, maintains an interpersonal order" (Levinas, 1969, p. 234). It is not with the nothingness of death, of which we are completely ignorant, that the analysis should begin, but, rather, within the context where something absolutely unknowable appears. It is this unknowableness of approaching death that becomes, in a certain sense, a knowable quality (Nemo, 1998, p. 50). "Death is the end of what makes the thinkable thinkable, and it is in this sense that it is unthinkable" (Levinas, 2000a, p. 90). An approaching death is thus a relation with something absolutely other, not something that we can fathom, assimilate, and make intelligible. It points to an interpersonal order, an unassimilable otherness, whose signification cannot be eradicated. It is precisely because death is not a merely an individual happening, but an interpersonal relation, that rescues it from absolute absurdity. In a word, "My solitude is thus not confirmed by death [as Heidegger thought] but broken by it" (Levinas, 1987, p. 74). In a certain sense, Levinas boldly says, it is impossible to annihilate oneself, nothingness is impossible, death is eternal mystery, ungraspable, unmasterable—"Death is never assumed, it comes" (*ibid.*, pp. 72–73). "It is an event without a project insofar as the 'project' that one might have of death is undone in the last moment" (Levinas, 2001a, p. 122). Thus, Levinas claims, suicide is a contradictory notion, in that while one can take life, one cannot take death, it is beyond one's capacities for self-assertion of the "I can", it cannot be assumed (Llewelyn, 1995, p. 10).

Waiting to die, in other words, requires great patience (and, ultimately, enforced passivity, the collapse of the will); this is "death understood as the patience of time" (Levinas, 2000a, p. 8). This is especially true if killing yourself is not an option. In my mother's case, though this was briefly considered, as I accidentally discovered when I found some Hemlock Society literature under the pillow of her favourite sitting chair, the fact is, as she told me, she did not have the courage to do herself in and did not want her children to have to cope with her exiting in such a violent way. Yet, it need not have been violent, but could have been done peacefully. Clearly, there remained a part of herself that clung to life, that had some flickering hope of a reprieve from her death sentence. "Time," says Levinas, "is pure hope. It is even the birthplace of hope" (Levinas, 2000a, p. 96). (In the case of my mother, following Shalom Aleichem, "hope was a liar".) Instead, my mother indicated that she had to "wait her turn" until the fateful hour occurred. This future not grasped, what would ultimately lay hold of her, is the relationship with the other (*ibid.*, p. 229). As far as she was concerned, an approaching death that allowed her to think the future (in the sense that while she was still alive, death was not with her) could not come fast enough. I remember once, it was *Kol Nidre* night and I stopped in to see her before going to synagogue, I asked my mother, who hardly knew that it was the night of Yom Kippur, and who was sitting by the window of her high-rise apartment watching the beautiful sunset, whether there was anything she wanted me to pray for, for her sake? Appearing almost completely coiled up within herself, her barely audible reply was, "Ask God to kill me quickly, tonight." As my mother was more or less an atheist, her comment, which I found shocking and deeply troubling at the time, illustrates well Levinas's idea that death is an engagement with an other; in this case, the other was not the straightforward sadistic adversary mentioned earlier, but rather the other whose sadism could possibly be taken advantage of and transformed into a kind of mercy killing. This, at least, was my mother's fantasy, a wilful effort at escape from her sense of impotent entrapment in the face of her capricious predator, whom she knew would choose the time and circumstance of her death.

To summarize: for my mother, her approaching death was an engagement with a violent, invisible adversary against whom she could not effectively retaliate; she was vulnerable to "absolute violence, to murder in the night" (Levinas, 1969, p. 233). This adversary could not be defeated by reason or will; in fact, as I will shortly discuss, approaching death fundamentally signifies the death of the will. Radical passivity in the face of an alien, sadistic power constitutes the consciousness of one's mortality. My point, following Levinas, is that death is not part of the relationship with the Self as usually understood, and thus cannot be comprehended or made intelligible in any ultimate way (contra Heidegger, it is not part of an "existential" or, as others' think, an "intentional" project). Rather, death lies permanently beyond experience, is utterly unknowable, and marks the end of the subject's mastery. This encounter with something outside the self, at least the self as it usually construes itself, is a relationship with the other as Mystery.

Perhaps it was my mother's experience of going to sleep at night, of "getting through the terrible nights," as she described them, that best suggests what this relationship with this menacing, mysterious other felt like. It was a form of suffering in which there was no refuge, "the fact of being directly exposed to being", and points to a main aspect of my mother's struggle with her physical illness and approaching death, "the impossibility of nothingness" (Levinas, 1987, p. 69). While my mother often spoke about feeling "nothingness", as it related to her dying, it is this ambiguity of death and its unknowability that I want to describe further.

First, it should be pointed out that there were medical reasons why the nights and, to a slightly lesser extent, the mornings, felt so awful for my mother, reasons that have to do with the trajectory of liver cancer. However, as my mother noted, though her suffering had physiological anchoring and manifestations (e.g., sweating, body pains, psychomotor agitation), there was a psychological overlay, including a disturbing dream life, that made the nights and the mornings feel even worse. Her insomnia and, ironically, her dread of awakening, both point to what Levinas called the "there is" anonymous or impersonal being that signifies "the impossibility of death". As Nemo pointed out in another context, "hell is not death; it is eternal life within suffering" (Nemo, 1998, p. 99).

Briefly, the "there is" is one of Levinas's most enigmatic philosophical abstractions, a kind of hypothetical construct, a "thought experiment" meant to evoke a dimension of being, of deeply internal experience, that is central to the Levinasian project. The notion of the "there is" is "elemental", a key notion that helps to animate Levinas's efforts to further his project of describing and explicating "how our encounter with the Other enters into the drama of consciousness" (Davis, 1996, p. 23). Levinas's notion of the "there is" attempts to describe the relationship between the burden of existing and the human Other that demands an ethical response.

According to Peperzak, Levinas believes that the "there is" is "a treacherous semblance of nothingness, a hiding place of mythical powers without face, an indeterminate and opaque density without orientation or meaning, a senseless and therefore terrifying chaos" (Peperzak, 1993, p. 163). The "there is", says Levinas, pre-exists nothingness, it is evoked in the terrifying silence facing the vigilant insomniac. The vigilant insomniac is and is not an "I" who cannot manage to fall asleep. This experience is not simply one of anxiety, at least not as conventionally conceived, even by psychoanalysts. Rather, it is something even more frightening and menacing, though Levinas only hints at this difference:

> The impossibility of escaping wakefulness is something "objective", independent of my initiative. This impersonality absorbs my consciousness; consciousness is depersonalized. I do not stay awake; "it" stays awake. Perhaps death is an absolute negation wherein "the music ends". . . . But in the maddening "experience" of the "there is" one has the impression of a total impossibility of escaping, of "stopping the music". [Levinas, 1985, p. 49]

The "there is", says Levinas, thus signifies the end of objectivizing consciousness, as it is not an object of perception or conscious thought and cannot be comprehended or intentionally created. According to him, it is impossible to avoid the experience of the "there is" because one is immersed and inundated in it. This inescapability, experienced as dread and panic, suggests Levinas, signifies "the impossibility of death . . . the impossibility of escaping from an anonymous and uncorruptible [*sic*] existence" (Levinas, 1989b, p. 33). This statement is similar to a feeling that my mother often described as "losing herself", as being lodged in a situation or state of being characterized by "supreme indetermination", without exit. One of her dreams sharply depicted this "impossibility of death", with its associated dread and panic.

My mother dreamt that she was under the ocean (remember that she loved the ocean, her symbol of peaceful nurturance), and she began to sense that she had no air and was drowning. Rather than panic, she felt accepting of it, and embraced the pleasant sensation, which, she said, was like the blissful anticipation of falling asleep after a long, productive, but exhausting day. As she was falling into a deeper sleep, she suddenly noticed her dead husband (my father, who had been dead for many years) floating away with a smile on his face. In what she described as her sudden change of feeling, she again became aware that she was drowning, only this time it was not peaceful, but terrifying, choking, and a gasping for air, a death-panic that just kept going without let-up. She woke up sweating, her chest pounding, and utterly unnerved. Her first response to the dream was that she did not understand why she did not simply drown peacefully, as in the first part of the dream, but rather dreamt of violently drowning. "Why couldn't I let go and just die?" she once asked me.

In our interpretation of her dream, and we only discussed it briefly for a few minutes before she received a telephone call, my mother felt that it expressed her wish that she would die quietly, symbolized by her peaceful drowning in the first part of the dream, and by her initial sense of wanting to join my dead, smiling father floating away. Then, for some unknown reason, the "good" drowning, as she called it, turned violent and panic-filled. She said that she did not know why she could not give way to a peaceful death, but then added a moment or two later, "Maybe I am guilty about something, maybe I did something wrong that required me to be punished . . . I often feel like I made a mess of my life sometimes." I tried, more as an anxious and overwhelmed son trying to "fix" things, to reduce her stinging self-judgement, than as an empathic, explorative psychoanalyst, "What person with any depth of thinking and honesty doesn't feel that they, in some sense, didn't mess their life up?" My mother intellectually agreed with my point, but appeared to be utterly unmoved by my words—"Don't wait for the Last Judgment," said Albert Camus, in *The Fall* (1991), "it is taking place every day".

What my mother could not escape, even in a make-believe death in her dream life, was the feeling that she was a moral failure in her relations with others and herself. As I mentioned in her eulogy, my mother told me that in her view her life "was all for naught", as she "had not been a good person and was a selfish phoney". Conscience, says Levinas, is the recognition of our obligations to the Other, to all Others. In my view, this includes, at least on a secondary level, the obligations to oneself, as Other. It is the mindfulness of the fact that my responsibilities are allocated to me to serve and care for others, and the awareness of the guilt of not having done so, or not nearly enough, that, along with making concrete efforts to "put things right", constitutes the proper operations of conscience in the Levinasian sense. My mother, being the harsh critic she was, at least at the time of her dream, judged herself as guilty. She had, in her view, failed to do enough for others, she was not a "good enough" wife, mother, grandmother, friend, or citizen. In addition, what made matters worse, she felt aware of her own selfishness and her need to use others to sustain herself, such as frequently "playing to the crowd", as she described it, but deceived herself into believing, at least at the time, that she was motivated otherwise. Such moments of self-understanding, of acknowledged "bad faith", as Sartre called it, can have a corrosive impact on one's resiliency as death approaches. It can also be redemptive, in that it can motivate one to be, and do, better, even as the end approaches. The responsible self is a judging self, it acknowledges itself as guilty, "the more I am just the more guilty I am" (Levinas, 1969, p. 244). In my mother's case, however, the fact that in her view she did not have the time or ability to put things right, not even to make meaningful reparations, further depressed her. Such an awareness of the irreversibility of lived time, that there is no going back, is a hard-to-swallow fact of existence that we all grapple with.

My mother's horror of the night was not merely anxiety about nothingness and the fear of death, as Heidegger and most psychoanalysts usually construe it. Rather, according to Levinas,

> there is horror of . . . the fact that tomorrow one still has to live, a tomorrow contained in the infinity of today. There is horror of immortality, perpetuity of the drama of existence, necessity of forever taking on his burden. [Levinas, 1989b, pp. 34–35]

Levinas is contrasting the horror of the night to Heideggerian anxiety, fear of being to Heideggerian fear of nothingness. The primordial anxiety and fear for Levinas is mere being, existing forever, with no escape, to be trapped in the nocturnal horror of existence that is prior to the emergence of consciousness. Perhaps it was this experience of the "there is" that my mother was facing each night, with all of its panic and horror, the impossibility of dying. Similarly, it was in the mornings, especially the first half hour after waking, when she felt most physically wretched, and realized that she was still alive and had to face the unbearable drudgery of what she took to be her anonymous existence. It was in these days, days without meaning or purpose, with only the passivity of an exposed subjectivity to the ambiguity of nothingness and the unknown of approaching death, that she uttered her most self-subverting and, for me, her most impossible-to-listen-to pained reflections. Indeed, at these unbearable moments, I often thought to myself that my mother was speaking to, and of, and from an irreducible and inexplicable transitional space, from a kind of awful twilight zone, an empty space located between being and nothingness, en route to somewhere or nowhere.

Death as a source of goodness

As I have suggested, following Levinas, my mother's encounter with her approaching death is best understood as "one of the modalities of the relationship with the Other", a modality characterized by radical alterity and originating and situated in the realm of mysterious and ungraspable murder (Levinas, 1969, p. 234). However, while such a formulation, in which approaching death is equated with an encounter with the Other as murderer, would seem to render one's death as pointless, if not absurd, Levinas indicates otherwise: "Death cannot drain all meaning from life" (*ibid.*, p. 236) because there is still time to be for the Other:

> The will ... on the way to death but a death ever future, exposed to death but not immediately, has time to be for the Other, and thus recover meaning despite death ... The goodness whose meaning death cannot efface, has its center outside itself. [Levinas, 1969 p. 236]

What Levinas is getting at is that the time that is left until one's death, at least theoretically, is enough time to do one last thing for the Other, one last act of kindness. It is this act (or acts) of giving and serving the Other, "this goodness liberated from the egoist gravitation" (*ibid.*), that will, in some sense, survive me. "To go beyond death is to sacrifice oneself. . . . I approach the Infinite by sacrificing myself" (Levinas, 1996a, p. 76). Such an other-directed and other-regarding act, which is radically opposed to the highly narcissistic nature of dying, creates an enduring meaning in the Other, one that does not end with my life, a meaning that the inevitability of my rapidly approaching death cannot eradicate. In this sense, and this was true with my mother, one is somehow able to live "beyond death", a kind of immortality for the non-believer. As I told my dying mother, the love we gave in our life we leave behind, and it endures; the love we received, we take with us.

Levinas's claim, that selfless being for the Other, which is what he means by goodness ("taking up a position in being such that the Other counts more than myself"), is the best antidote to the sting of dying is probably more of an ideal than a compelling reality for most people. In the case of my mother, and I believe this is fairly common, as she became sicker and sicker, she became less and less interested in the external world and more self-centred, her coma being the final indicator of this inward seclusion, this shut-upness. Indeed, it is a frequent observation that a dying person usually becomes progressively more inner-directed, burrowing into the self, as she prepares to give up the outside world and begin "the journey home", as they say in the hospice world. Though my mother did not make any grand gestures of being for the Other during the three months before she died, the fact is that she did to a number of small things that support Levinas's claim. For example, she made certain that her financial affairs were in perfect order and that all three of her children knew that everything was divided evenly among the three of them; she left considerable money to each of her grandchildren, to be used only for their education; she spoke to her grandchildren and affirmed that what they had chosen to do with their work lives, though somewhat unorthodox in the case of my children, was praiseworthy. "You must be willing to risk everything to fulfil your dream," she told my daughter, an aspiring actress; she stressed over and over that once she died she wanted her children always to remain loyal and supportive to each other, that it was an unrefuseable obligation to each other; she affirmed to all three of her children that she was proud of what we had accomplished in our work and personal lives; she emphasized to her children that we should not let her death shatter our lives, that it was entirely in the nature of things that she moves on and we move on; most importantly, at least in terms of my relationship with my mother—a woman towards whom I often felt ambivalent, whom I often felt was the source of much of my own psychic pain over the years, and whom I had often felt never really deeply cherished me—was the fact that her last coherent and intended words to me before she lapsed into a coma were words that put things right, her last and most precious "gift" to me: she looked into my eyes, gently caressed my cheek, and said, "I love you."

This experience of love, expressed in speech, reveals that through the Other one can overcome temporal death or, rather, one can live beyond it. Indeed, death can nurture love, it can evoke the commanding power of love, conceived as responsibility for the Other, as it did in my mother and in me. As Levinas noted, the essence of responsibility for the Other is manifested in how one responds to the Other in their suffering and approaching death: "Death . . . is present only in the Other, and only in him does it summon me urgently to my final essence, to my responsibility" (Levinas, 1969, p. 179). In other words, it was my encounter with my mother in her suffering and approaching death that evoked in me and my siblings the "call to giving and serving", "to not let the Other alone", and, even more poignantly, to not let her "die alone", as Levinas puts it. "The fear for the death of the other is certainly at the basis of the responsibility for him" (Levinas, 1985, p. 119). Put in more straightforward psychological terms, we can say that "the other individuates me in the responsibility I have for him" (Levinas, 2000a, p. 12).

This notion that the suffering of the Other evokes in the witness an unavoidable and unsubstitutable responsibility to tend to him was experienced by me and my siblings in a number of very concrete ways as it relates to my mother, ways that are familiar to most adult children in similar circumstances: such common actions as visiting and calling her regularly, sleeping over at her apartment when she was feeling most vulnerable and alone, arranging for and closely monitoring her companion care, taking her to doctors and helping her keep track of her medicines and insurance forms, helping her with cooking and cleaning and the like, and, in my case, speaking with her about herself, helping her to make peace with herself as she prepared to exit, to help her as she did her final "life review", as Erik Erikson said, with a sense of integrity rather than despair. The meaningfulness of my mother's "face", conceived as her defencelessness, helplessness, her naked exposure to death, was the command of responsibility for her that it evoked in her children.

There is an aspect of the experience of tending to a suffering and dying mother that is sometimes overlooked, an obscured aspect that a Levinasian sensibility may help put into sharper focus. It pertains to what was common between my mother's suffering as she lay dying and my suffering as I watched her slip away.

> There is a radical difference between *the suffering in the other*, where it is unforgivable to *me*, solicits me and calls me, and suffering *in me*, my own experience of suffering, whose constitutional or congenital uselessness can take on a meaning, the only one of which suffering is capable, in becoming a suffering for suffering . . . of someone else. [Levinas, 1998a, p. 94]

In other words, both my mother's suffering, and my suffering for her suffering (and they are not existentially equivalent), were in a certain sense "useless," meaningless, and insurmountable, to the extent that each remained located in the realm of solitude. Suffering experienced only as a private matter, as "a question of perceiving oneself locked within a self-preoccupation, a self-enclosed ego or state of narcissism", is "useless suffering", as Levinas famously wrote (O'Connor, 1961, p. 230). In contrast, when my mother and I construed our suffering as a problem of responsibility for the Other, the suffering assumed a kind of self-transcendent meaning, one that went beyond the "savage malignancy" of, for example, her physical pain and my psychic pain. Put somewhat differently, all pain and suffering (and they are not exactly equivalent) undermines the self-encapsulation, self-sufficiency, narcissism, and autonomy of the self, especially the conquering, mastery-orientated "virility of being" I described earlier. Such undermining of the virile self puts the sufferer in touch with a fundamental feature of pain and suffering, which is that, to some extent, all pain is inherently interhuman.

Whether it is the drill of the dentist, or facing suffering and approaching death, or, as in my case, witnessing the latter, the sufferer pleads for relief from his suffering, and this almost always involves wishing for the helping and nurturing hand of a caring and compassionate other. "Death approaches in the . . . hopes in someone" (Levinas, 1969, p. 234). My mother did not want to die alone, despite what she sometimes said, she wanted the comfort and support of her children even though, at times, she could not let our love in. Likewise, it was for this reason that my mother's final "gift" to me—caressing my cheek and telling me she loved me—was so moving; it was her way of compassionately caring for me, of being for the Other. Levinas aptly makes this point in his analysis of the caress as it relates to physical pain, though his observation has more general relevance, especially for the psychoanalyst or psychotherapist whose job it is to care for the suffering analysand:

> The caress of a consoler [e.g., the kind and insightful words of the analyst], which softly comes in our pain does not promise the end of suffering, does not announce any compensation, and in its very contact, is not concerned with what is to come with afterwards in *economic* time; it concerns the very instant of physical [and psychological] pain, which is then no longer condemned to itself, is transported "elsewhere" by the movement of the caress, and is freed from the vice-grip of "oneself", finds "fresh air", a dimension and a future. [Levinas, 2001b, p. 93]

By compassionately embracing the other's pain and suffering, as I did my mother's and she did mine, a form of consolation we gave freely, we release the sufferer from his agonizing isolation and solitude. We release the suffering Other from her feeling of being trapped in a maze of grotesque happenings, at least to some extent. Through our caring words and deeds we give the sufferer the beginning of a way out, a measure of relief and hope that, mercifully, there is a light at the end of the tunnel, there is hope, however that is construed by the person. One way or the other, perhaps for just a moment, the sufferer feels the liberating effect of our unconditional giving, serving, and solidarity with his pain and suffering, and in my mother's case, her approaching death. "Please hold my hand," my mother unexpectedly whispered to me during a conversation, no doubt during an unbearable wave of fear and forlornness.

Thus, following Levinas, my claim is that what most of us, including psychoanalysts, have not adequately appropriated into our thinking about pain, suffering, and approaching death, is the "usefulness" of helping the sufferer give meaning to his suffering by developing an ethical response to it, one that is for the Other. Whether it is my, or the other's suffering, or the suffering that my suffering causes the other, the way to make such suffering "sufferable", at least in general terms, is to perceive it as an ethical problem requiring an other-directed, other-regarding response. Such an ethical response is an asymmetrical and non-reciprocal responsibility to and for the Other, whether another person, or one's God, or its secular equivalent. As the rabbis of the Talmud noted in their discussion of the need for the humanitarian treatment of an enemy, and Levinas would no doubt agree with this as it pertains to the individual facing suffering and death, "the greatest hero . . . is he who changes his enemy into a friend". That is, the surest way of becoming most fully human is to transform the "enemy", that is, suffering and approaching death, by acts of loving kindness.

CHAPTER FOUR

On reading a sacred book: the wisdom of Ecclesiastes and its significance for psychoanalysis*

> "Yes, I perceived that this, too, is chasing after wind. For the more wisdom, the more grief, and increasing one's knowledge means increasing one's pain"
>
> Ecclesiastes

This chapter explores one of the most profound, subversive, and beautiful books in the Hebrew Bible, Ecclesiastes, known as Koheleth ("member of the assembly") in Hebrew. The author of Ecclesiastes does not present a consistently thought-out system or logical structure in his reflections; rather, in his brief talks, parables, maxims, and proverbs we are presented with a series of free associations on the meaning of existence, the good that people can achieve in life, and the problems inherent in attaining or creating an enduring sense of personal happiness. Specifically, Ecclesiastes contains the melancholy, sceptical, ironic, and rationalist reflections

*Earlier versions of this essay appeared in the *Psychoanalytic Review* (2000) and my book, *Ancient Religious Wisdom, Spirituality and Psychoanalysis* (2003).

of a philosopher–poet at the sunset of his life rather than a straightforward, unambivalent, pious affirmation of faith and the virtues of living an exacting religious life. Not only does Ecclesiastes strongly question some of the core beliefs in Jewish tradition and its world-view, but, most importantly for this chapter, he raises many profound questions about human experience and the course of life, which have been of concern to most serious thinkers for thousands of years and, more recently, to psychoanalysts and others in the so-called mental health professions.

My claim in this chapter is that, as one of the most illustrious of the "Wisdom" writers—those ancient professional teacher sages who were committed to developing "a realistic approach to the problems of life, including the practical skills and the technical arts of civilization" (Gordis, 1951, pp. 16–17)—Ecclesiastes not only identifies with startling brilliance and poetic insight some of the central problems of the human condition as modern man construes it, but offers what is in many ways a reasonable and feasible attitude towards contemporary life. Moreover, Ecclesiastes' way of looking at life is similar to certain life attitudes and values embodied implicitly in the Freudian world-view, but also suggests what psychoanalysis might, in part, appropriate or further explore and develop as it tries to enhance itself as a narrative of the human condition and a compelling "technology of the self". In other words, Ecclesiastes provides us with some of the most illuminating and insightful reflections on modern existence and our sense of what, for many, ultimately matters in life. Psychoanalysis, as it is concerned with the "arts of living" the "good life", can only benefit from an engagement with the at times angst-ridden but always fearless truth-seeker and lover of life from Jerusalem.

Who was Ecclesiastes?

There is a vast and divergent scholarly literature on Ecclesiastes. Both the more sceptical and the pious have found support for their preferred interpretation (e.g., Bickerman, 1967; Crenshaw, 1987; Ginsberg, 1969; Gordis, 1951; Perry, 1993; Zlotowitz, 1996). Briefly, as Gordis (1951)—in my view, the seminal scholar on Ecclesiastes—has noted, the Book of Ecclesiastes was written in Hebrew by a Jew residing in Jerusalem, who knew Aramaic but no Greek, though he was knowledgeable about certain Greek ideas such as the "golden mean" (pp. 22, 68, 78). The book was written toward the end of Ecclesiastes' life, about 250 BCE, which corresponded with the experience of national defeat, humiliation, and subjugation, between about the fifth to the second centuries. Scholars have inferred that Ecclesiastes was probably something of a country gentleman, a bachelor with no children who probably came from a comfortable upper middle-class background with a socially and politically conservative outlook. The tradition of the Synagogue, however, assumes (Zlotowitz, 1996), incorrectly, according to most scholars (Ginsberg, 1999), that it was none other than Solomon, the son of David, who wrote the Book of Ecclesiastes. This view is, in part, based on the opening verse, in which Ecclesiastes introduces himself as Solomon: "The Words of Koheleth, son of David, King in Jerusalem". However, most scholars believe that Koheleth is using a literary convention. That is, maintains Gordis (1951), he is impersonating Solomon because he wants to demonstrate that both wisdom and pleasure arc meaningless as goals in life, and Solomon was well known to have had an abundance of both. To further complicate matters, the name Koheleth, translated as "convener" or "gatherer", is in the Hebrew feminine form, thereby implying a female author (Cohen, 2000).

As I have said, Ecclesiastes was one of the professional teachers of Hebrew Wisdom, one manifestation of the literary genre that was part of the social world of the Fertile Crescent, which existed in Egypt, Babylonia, Syria, and Palestine during the second and first millennia BCE (Gordis, 1951, p. 9). Ecclesiastes probably taught in one of the well-to-do local academies that educated upper-class Jewish youth. Wisdom literature is the most secular branch of ancient Hebrew literature, compared to Torah (with its focus on the practical and exacting obligations of living a pious and God-fearing life) and Prophecy (which focused on the ethical perfection of the Jewish nation and social justice). Wisdom, as Scott (1965) has pointed out, in general "taught a practical philosophy through which a good man might find satisfaction in life, in a moral order which had established itself through experience" (p. xvii).

Although Hebrew Wisdom had its antecedents in more ancient cultures (e.g., Egypt, Phoenicia, and Mesopotamia) and neighbouring groups (e.g., Edomites), there are basically two main kinds of Wisdom literature, which embodied the contrasting attitudes among the Jewish sages (Scott, 1965, pp. xviii, xix). The first is exemplified in the Bible by the Book of Proverbs. It tends to be conservative, pragmatic, didactic, optimistic, and worldly wise. The second type is highly critical, almost rebellious, in its attitude towards traditional beliefs. This second type of Wisdom literature tends to be theoretical, individualistic, and pessimistic. Ecclesiastes, like Job, is in this second group. The former sought a rational comprehension of human existence and a foundation for ethics through the use of logic and critical reason to observable data and experience (*ibid.*, p. 196).

While Ecclesiastes believed in God (though not exactly the conventional God of his time), for it was inconceivable at that time for a Jew to believe otherwise, his focus as a Wisdom teacher was on the problems of individual existence and experience. He addresses the difficulties of creating an existentially tolerable if not meaningful life and attaining a degree of personal happiness, all within the context of certain deeply troubling "facts" of human existence, such as the transitory nature of life, the certainty of death, and man's sense of helplessness before an ultimately unfathomable and uncontrollable universe. Ecclesiastes, like Freud, is characterized by his unshakable intellectual integrity, his courageous use of reason in facing the most agonizing problems of life, his absolute refusal of sureness where he saw ambiguity and uncertainty, and his relentless devotion to truth, regardless of the uncomfortable ramifications in one's personal life (Gordis, 1951, pp. 37–38). Moreover, like Freud, Ecclesiastes was attempting to reconfigure his subjectivity, to fashion a self as an autonomous and self-governing being, both within the context of the parameters of the society he lived in, and in terms of what he took to be the limitations inherent in Being (and in Ecclesiastes' case, in terms of the seeming limitations and enigmas in God's relationship to man). Finally, like Freud at his best, Ecclesiastes was committed to a relentless critique of himself and his world as his main mode of self-fashioning. Ecclesiastes questioned nearly all of the social paradigms and interpretations of self that were operative in his time, and in this sense he was, to some extent, attempting to fashion a new form of life that departed from the coercive normalizing institutions of the priestly scribes and orthodox theologians within his community. Finally, as I will suggest, like Freud, Ecclesiastes ended up, in part, advocating an attitude towards life characterized by resignation without despair, combined with an unwavering commitment to striving after joy in life, fleeting as these joyful experiences may be.

The Book of Ecclesiastes is overflowing with provocative ideas about life, love, suffering, growing old, and death, and it is impossible in this chapter to discuss all of them. Therefore, I focus on a few of the major themes that embody his "philosophy of life", as it were, and that seem to be most relevant to psychoanalysis. In the final section, I discuss the implications for psychoanalysis of Ecclesiastes' insights into the human condition and the ethical wisdom that emanates from it.

"Vanity of vanities, all is vanity" (or "chasing after wind")

From beginning to end, Ecclesiastes bluntly asserts one of his recurring claims, that from his wide-ranging experience of life, the entire human enterprise is fundamentally empty and ultimately meaningless:

> Vanities of vanities, says Koheleth, vanities of vanities, all is vanity [in Hebrew *hebel*, translated as "vanity", means "vapour" or "breath"]. What profit has a man of all his toil beneath the sun? [i.e., the earthly context of man's activities and vicissitudes]. One generation goes and another comes, but the earth is forever unchanged. The sun rises and the sun sets, breathlessly rushing towards the place where it is to rise again. Going to the south and circling to the north, the wind goes round and round, and then returns its tracks. All the rivers flow into the sea, but the sea is never full; to the place where the rivers flow, there they continue to flow. All things are tiresome, one cannot put them into words, and so the eye is never satisfied with seeing nor the ear filled with hearing. What has been will be, and what has been done will be done again; there is nothing new under the sun. There may be something of which man says, 'Look, this is new!' It has already occurred in the ages before us [including the musings of Koheleth!] For there is no recollection left of the earliest generations, and even the later ones will not be remembered who come at the very end. [1: 2–11, translated by Gordis, 1951, p. 136]

Ecclesiastes is here declaring his key conviction about life, that man's existence, his experience of his life's struggles and all that he attempts to achieve, is like a vapour or a breath. Like nature, we are part of a repetitive and eternal cycle, without an endpoint or inherent purpose. Nothing really new ever happens; our experience of our life is of an endless movement without change. What appears to be new is actually a function of our truncated memory, that is, we forget the past. Thus, as the famous quotation goes, "there is nothing new under the sun". From this perspective of the universe, concludes Ecclesiastes, all man's efforts are pointless. That man can neither fully comprehend nor modify the predetermined pattern of life is most beautifully expressed in the famous Catalogue of the Times (popularized by the rock group, The Byrds):

> Everything has its appointed time, and there is a season for every event under the sky.
> There is a time to be born, and a time to die,
> A time to plant and a time to uproot,
> A time to kill and a time to heal.
> A time to wreck and a time to build.
> A time to weep and a time to laugh,
> A time to mourn and a time to dance,
> A time to scatter stones and a time to gather them,
> A time to embrace and a time to hold off embraces.
> A time to seek and a time to give up.
> A time to keep and a time to cast off, A time to tear and a time to repair,
> A time to be silent and a time to speak.
> A time to love and a time to hate,
> A time of war and a time of peace.
> What profit then has the worker in his toil?
>
> [III: 1–15, translated by Gordis, 1951, p. 144]

In Ecclesiastes' view, all that happens to man seems to be predetermined, and correlated to its uniquely apt time. However, why it occurs this way and not in some different way, and what it all means (if anything) is an unfathomable enigma (Scott, 1965, pp. 202–203). Ecclesiastes never resolves the contradiction to which all determinists are vulnerable. That is, Ecclesiastes was assuming man's freedom of choice in terms of the practical attitudes and conduct he was recommending, yet he claims that all is predetermined by God (Gordis, 1951, p. 55). I think that Ecclesiastes was advocating resigned submission to the order of the world, yet also encouraging man not to be passive. In other words, in a limited sense, man has freedom of action as well as a choice between different courses of action (Cohen, 1970, p. 154).

In the preceding interpretation of Ecclesiastes, the analogy between the processes of nature and human experience illustrates that life proceeds in an endless repetition that is always a negative force. Some scholars, however, have interpreted this passage differently, as suggesting a less pessimistic side to Ecclesiastes. Perry (1993, pp. 14–21), for example, notes that while it appears that man is part of nature and thus subject to its causality, and that the direction of life is irreversible, from positive to negative (e.g., "the sun rises and the sun sets", "a time to be born, a time to die"), Ecclesiastes also is aware of the counterpoint, and here, perhaps, lies his tepid optimism. That is, the "alternative to natural determinism and pessimism", says Perry, is a "concept of cyclicality" such that following decline, deterioration, and death there is a new beginning. For example, despite its previous setting, the sun always rises again. In other words, continues Perry, while Ecclesiastes seems to be saying on one hand, that endless repetition is negative, the notion of cyclicality, which can be negative or positive, opens the possibility of trying again. Moreover, says Perry, in the human context, many of the verses in the Catalogue of Times actually insinuate hopefulness and optimism, for example, "A time to weep but also a time to be happy". While I agree with Perry that both pessimism and to some extent a restrained optimism are woven into Ecclesiastes' reflections, I believe the pessimism is the much stronger voice, for good reason according to how Ecclesiastes construes the workings of the harsh world.

How does Ecclesiastes know that life is fundamentally futile, that is, what does he base his assertion on? He bases it on two forms of personal experimentation in giving meaning to existence—one broadly philosophical–intellectual and the other sensual—both of which are entirely contemporary, but which Ecclesiastes, have failed him as a satisfying justification for his existence:

> I, Koheleth, was king over Israel in Jerusalem. I applied my mind to search out and explore in my wisdom all that happens beneathe the sky—a sorry business it is that God has given men to be

> afflicted with . . . . Said I to myself, "Here I have greatly increased my wisdom, beyond all those who were before me over Jerusalem, for my heart has attained much wisdom and knowledge." But as I applied my mind, I learnt that wisdom [equivalent to "perfect goodness" for the Wisdom writers, asserts Gordis, 1951, p. 268] and knowledge are madness [unrestrained and unprincipled behaviour rooted in the belief that life is meaningless and there is no moral law working in the everyday world; Gordis, 1951, p. 291] and folly. Yes, I perceived that this, too, is chasing after wind. For the more wisdom, the more grief, and increasing one's knowledge means increasing one's pain.
>
> Then I said to myself, "Come let me try you out in joy and enjoy pleasure", but this, too, was vanity. Of laughter I said, "It is folly", and of joy, "What good is it?" For I had explored the manner with my mind, by stimulating my body with wine (while my mind was acting with wisdom) and by taking hold of frivolity, so that I might see what course is best for men under the sky during the brief span of their lives. [I: 12–II. 3, translated by Gordis, 1951, pp. 138, 140]

Ecclesiastes is here noting that God has lodged in man an irrepressible desire to find the Truth, to make some ultimate sense out of life by imposing an all-embracing, comprehensive order and a system on his experience. That is, Ecclesiastes is making the profound deconstructionist point that any attempt to frame a complete, totalizing, philosophical system can be achieved only by doing violence to an ultimately unfathomable reality. In other words, in religious language, "What God is doing is his own secret and whether He is well-disposed or ill-disposed toward man is unknown" (Scott, 1965, p. 198). While man's desire to find the Truth is compelling, according to Ecclesiastes this is impossible, and the humbler search for usable truths is the best we can do. Truth, for Ecclesiastes, is, thus, roughly equated with a pragmatic outlook in which finding "workable" solutions to the problems of existence is the main criterion. Moreover, Ecclesiastes ironically notes, the quest for and attainment of knowledge and wisdom (or "insight" as psychoanalysts call it) can lead to more psychic pain. In a sense, ignorance is bliss, although Ecclesiastes clearly values knowledge and wisdom above ignorance, foolishness, and madness—but not by much!

Ecclesiastes also says that he tried to derive enduring meaning in his life largely through the attainment of sensual pleasure, for example, in the form of wine, women, song, wealth, and possessions. That this gratification of the appetites, pleasure for its own sake, ultimately left him feeling unsatisfied is not surprising, because, as Ecclesiastes notes, these acquisitions are even more transient and ephemeral in the long run than knowledge and wisdom. This is especially the case as one gets older, when one's bodily responsiveness to pleasurable stimulation is diminished and when one tends to quickly habituate to one's once novel pleasures.

Thus, Ecclesiastes' main claim is that experience—including its intellectual and sensual aspects—is as fleeting and insubstantial as a vapour. The evidence for this, in part, he claims, is that generations come and go and nature is in endless motion, but nothing new results. Human effort and so-called achievement is pointless, whether it is to change the world (for example, to fight for social justice as the prophets did was pointless because nothing changes; there is nothing new under the sun), to reach understanding (that is, man is forever ignorant of the "real" meaning of events; life is an insolvable enigma because God chooses not to reveal Himself), or to attain happiness (that is, man has a God-given "design fault"; he is never really satisfied no matter how much he acquires) (May & Metzger, 1973, p. 805).

If this is not a grim enough characterization of the human condition, Ecclesiastes adds other observations from his experience to support his pessimistic outlook:

> Furthermore, I saw under the sun that in the place of judgment there was wickedness, and in the place of righteousness, wrong. . . . Again I saw all the acts of oppression that are done under the sun. Here are the tears of the oppressed, with none to comfort them; and power in the hands of their oppressors, with none to comfort them. So I praise the dead who already have died, more than the creatures who still are alive. And more fortunate than both is he who has not yet been born and so has never seen the evil deeds that are being done under the sun. [III: 16, 1–3, translated by Gordis, 1951, p. 148]

Ecclesiastes' sense of the fundamental meaninglessness and inscrutability of life is further elaborated through his pained observation that there appears to be no divine or human justice in the world (in contrast, for example, to what the prophets believed).

Ecclesiastes was struck by the fact that, time and again, according to his experience, it is as if man lives in an ethically indifferent universe. Ecclesiastes believed that there was a God who had creative and boundless power, but that He often did not wish to intervene in human history at the appropriate time, or, if He did intervene, it was usually too little, too late. Ecclesiastes, thus, passionately protests against a world in which the powerful are evil and the weak vulnerable to victimization. He sees no evidence for, or comfort in, a belief in the Hereafter where the wicked will be punished and/or everything will be put right (a commonly held view in his day).

Perhaps even more outrageous to Ecclesiastes is that man's character, behaviour, and achievements appear to make no difference to his everyday or ultimate fate in this world. The righteous and the wicked, the wise man and the fool end up about the same, and both meet the same inevitable end, death. In fact, he somewhat sardonically notes, it is all too common for the righteous and wise to suffer and the wicked and foolish to prosper. Moreover, he claims that it is impossible for a man to know whether God will act kindly toward him, thus emphasizing a most tragic aspect to life, that man is uncertain of his fate. In fact, Ecclesiastes even sarcastically questions whether man is superior to the animal, because it is uncertain whether his spirit ascends to Heaven and the animal's descends to the earth (Scott, 1965, p. 203).

It is in his final reflection, in his magisterial "Allegory on old age", that Ecclesiastes describes how man gradually but decisively deteriorates physically and dies; Ecclesiastes puts into sharp focus the brevity and tragic limitations of existence. For this reason, and because it suggests what he thought was the most workable attitude toward life given his stark and pessimistic view (discussed in the next section), it is worth quoting the Allegory in its entirety (there have been many interpretations of this allegory based on Talmudic and other sources. I have mainly drawn from Cohen [1970] and Ginzberg [1969] for my parenthetical entries):

Sweet is the light [read: "life"; Scott, 1965, p. 183]
And it is good for the eyes
To see the sun! [read: "life"; *ibid.*]
For if a man lives many years,

Let him rejoice in them all,
And remember that the days of darkness will be many,
And that everything thereafter is nothingness.

Rejoice, young man, in your youth,
And let your heart cheer you in your youthful days.
Follow the impulses of your heart
And the desires of your eyes,
And know that for all this,
God will call you to account.

Banish sadness from your heart,
And remove sorrow from your flesh,
For childhood and youth are a fleeting breath.
Remember your Creator in the days of your youth,
Before the evil days come and the years draw near,
Of which you will say, "I have no pleasure in them."

Before the sun [the forehead] grows dark,
And the light [the nose] of the moon [the soul] and the stars [the cheeks],
And the clouds return after the rain [enfeebled eyesight due to trouble and sickness]

In the day when the watchman of the house [the flanks, ribs, arms] tremble,
And the strong men [the legs] are bent.
The grinding maidens [the teeth] cease, for they are few,
And the ladies peering through the lattices [the eyes] grow dim.

When the doubled doors on the street [the ears] are shut,
And the voice of the mill [a failing stomach] becomes low.
One wakes at the sound of a bird,
And all the daughters of song are laid low.
When one fears to climb a height,
And terrors lurk in a walk.
When the almond-tree blossoms [the whitening of the hair],

The grasshopper becomes a burden [the decline of sexual vitality].
And the caperberry [a sensual fruit] can no longer stimulate desire.
So man goes to his eternal home,
While the hired mourners walk about in the street. . . .

Before the silver cord [the tongue or the spine] is severed,
And the golden bowl [the marrow or the head] is shattered,
The pitcher [the gall or the stomach] is broken at the spring,

And the wheel [the skull] is shattered at the pit.
The dust returns to the earth as it was,
And the spirit returns to God, who gave it.
Vanities of vanities, says Koheleth, all is vanity.
[XI. 9–XII. 8, translated by Gordis, 1951, pp. 186, 188]

For Ecclesiastes, man's awareness that the time and context of his death are unknown adds to his sense of uncertainty and helplessness in a fundamentally unintelligible universe. Ecclesiastes ironically notes that as man's life draws to its absolute conclusion after a long and decisive period of deterioration, this tragedy is but a professional routine practice for the hired mourners, thus emphasizing that the vanity of life is mirrored and culminated in the vanity of death (Gordis, 1951, p. 337). Death, for Ecclesiastes, means that all activity is ended, although, as Gordis notes, he "does not deny that life comes from God" (p. 339). However, while Ecclesiastes' God is conceived of as real and transcendent, as the creator of the physical universe and of man, and as ruling over the course of events over the world, divine intervention in nature or human affairs is impossible because nothing new happens under the sun. Thus, the doctrine of divine Providence, a core belief in traditional Judaism, has become, for Ecclesiastes, an arbitrary, capricious and absolute determinism (Scott, 1965, p. 198). Says Gordis (1951, p. 339), "Before the mystery of death, only the language of religion proves adequate. But Koheleth does not conceive of God as Comforter or Redeemer", unlike the ancient Hebrews of his time. I would add, however, that Ecclesiastes did not view God as a Punisher, as the prophets did.

Last, says Ecclesiastes, just as life is depleted of its meaning by death, so all values are undermined, if not blotted out, by their opposites. For example, knowledge and wisdom often cause more psychic conflict and pain; things of great value or quality are frequently destroyed by some seemingly preordained, yet inexplicable, bad happening or disaster; frequently men do not acknowledge or affirm good deeds or wisdom, rendering them ineffective; capricious power is often in the hands of wicked people, causing much anguish to others and social instability; a famous and/or good man is frequently forgotten; and the hard-earned achievements and acquisitions of a lifetime may be destroyed or lost through one crucial mistake in judgment (Scott, 1965, p. 203). All values and the reality that they reflect are here dialectically conceived, implying that there is no absolute ethical foundation in which one can anchor one's life.

This is a summary of the way the world looks to Ecclesiastes. It is a rather grim view of life; as one commentator noted, "all this sounds like an argument for suicide" (Scott, 1965, p. 203). However, this is absolutely not Ecclesiastes' conclusion. The rest of this chapter will explain what the world-view and ethical wisdom of Ecclesiastes has to do with psychoanalysis, and, specifically, in what ways his "Freud-friendly" form of life and technology of the self can possibly enhance the psychoanalytic one.

The significance of Ecclesiastes' ethical wisdom for psychoanalysis

Ecclesiastes' philosophy of life is in part rooted in the conviction that it is unwise, if not impossible, to impose a comprehensive order and system, a worldview, on experience (e.g., the philosophical–intellectual and sensual-based approaches described earlier). For to do so is to distort experience by, for example, reducing it to comfortable and banal formulas that do not do justice to the complexity, ambiguity, and contradictory character of experience. For Ecclesiastes, the experience of life cannot be reduced to a totalizing system by means of moral principles because they collapse amidst the anomalies of experience, just as the attempt to reduce life to system by means of theoretical ideas collapses as it tries to resolve the antinomies, ironies, and paradoxes of existence (Guthrie & Motyer, 1970, p. 575). In other words, as Levinas has suggested, man seems to have a basic tendency to totalize individual experience by presuming either that the world is completely for him, or that the infinite (i.e., for Levinas, something-outside-and-beyond-everything, the Other, God) can actually be captured and encapsulated by individual experience, ideas, and conceptualizations. Ecclesiastes is thus brought to reincorporate "such pseudototalities into the infinite . . . by the conclusion that God is to be feared" (Perry, 1993, pp. 27–28), that is, God operates according to what appears to humans as an arbitrary, capricious, and absolute determinism. In this sense, the man of faith is more open-minded than the classical secular man of experience because the former, unlike the latter, is steadfastly "unwilling to foreclose on God's nature or to infer the nature of things in general from particular human" experiences (*ibid.*, p. 35). The man of faith, thus, relinquishes the urge to pin things down and put them firmly and permanently in their place.

Such a view, one that is against imposing an all-embracing system and order on experience, is congruent with the best of psychoanalysis. As Alan Bass (1998, pp. 412–413, cited in an editor's introduction by Marcus) has pointed out, Freud was against the idea of a psychoanalytic "worldview" (*Weltanschauung*), in part because it was anti-psychoanalytic, that is, it went against the basic thrust of psychoanalysis, which means for Bass, following Freud, that "it cannot be systematic". Philosophers, theologians, and psychotics, according to Freud, strive for systematicity, but psychoanalysis should not do so because it fundamentally concerns itself, says Bass, with "unconscious energic processes" that, by definition, are contradictory, paradoxical, and ambiguous, and, therefore, must challenge our habitual conscious patterns of organizing data and thinking about its meaning. (In Ecclesiastes' time this meant, for example, challenging the received wisdom of the priestly scribes and orthodox theologians.)

In other words, for Bass, like Freud (and Ecclesiastes), to seek out or create a world-view is to succumb to an "illusory wish fulfilment". Ecclesiastes says that man

> cannot discover the meaning of God's work which is done under the sun, for the sake of which a man may search hard, but he will not find it, and though a wise man may think he is about to learn it, he will be unable to find it. [VIII: 10–14,17, translated by Gordis, 1951, p. 176]

A commitment to such systematization is not only a form of imprisonment, but also misses some of the essential things about psychoanalysis that suggest what Freud (and Ecclesiastes) thought constituted important aspects of the human condition: for example, that human consciousness is unavoidably and undeniably ambiguous, contradictory, paradoxical, and fluid.

It is thus impossible and perhaps misguided to attempt to systematize Freudian psychoanalysis, whether as a theoretician or practitioner. Rather, Bass suggests, psychoanalysis (and, Ecclesiastes would say, one's attitude toward life) must push against the tendency to mould and shape itself into the habitual and familiar patterns of conscious perception; that is, it must push against world-views, striving to be more like an endless movement that perpetually undoes itself (says Ecclesiastes, "all the rivers flow into the sea, but the sea is never full; to the place where the rivers f1ow, there they continue to flow" [I: 2–11, 7, translated by Gordis, 1951, p. 136]).

While maintaining an anti-systematicity assumption, Ecclesiastes does, nevertheless, suggest that some attitudes towards life tend to be more useful than others. Thus, he offers some helpful, practical, experientially based attitudes towards existence that are strikingly compatible with a Freudian perspective. Both theoretical and clinical psychoanalysis can benefit from being more cognizant of these attitudes, as psychoanalysis both articulates its interesting and illuminating psychoanalytic story ("one good story—among many others—about what we are and who we want to be") and strives to help people achieve a greater degree of happiness amid their predicaments (Phillips, 1998, p. 24). In the spirit of Ecclesiastes' dialogic, open, pluralistic, and non-authoritarian intellectual and spiritual approach to truth, reality, and meaning (Perry, 1993, pp. 6–7), these attitudinal suggestions I describe represent some of the usable truths Ecclesiastes sought, as opposed to the absolute Truth that cannot be found.

Throughout his experience-guided discourse, Ecclesiastes asserts or implies that one must face the painful and distressing facts of life, that is, one must not continue to accept as true that which does not hold up to critical evaluation, to the evidence, so to speak, and, most importantly, to one's lived experience (Scott, 1965, p. 204). Ecclesiastes notes, for instance, that to the orthodox theologians and priestly scribes of his day, it was believed that the righteous will be rewarded in this life and the wicked will be punished. However, experience indicated to him that this is frequently not the case. Moreover, Ecclesiastes says that it is simply false that a commitment to wisdom and goodness, or the striving after pleasure, or the hoarding of wealth and material possessions adds up to sustained, solid, or permanent happiness.

For the psychoanalyst, this idea that one must face so-called facts and act accordingly is roughly similar to Freud's commitment to, and advocacy of, facing up to the hard truths about one's life even if the consequences are deeply disturbing. This idea speaks to what is at the heart of psychoanalysis. Continuing to assert so-called irrational and unreasonable convictions, to allow them to have a strong interpretative grip on one's life, is to succumb to neurosis. For example, the analysand who insists that his compulsive rituals and obsessive thinking actually protect him from external, real-life catastrophe is plainly not facing up to the evidence concerning the workings of the world. And the analysand who claims that having three consecutive marriages to men who turn out to be alcoholic is a sign of how defective contemporary men are in general, rather than accepting that it is she who unconsciously seeks out and chooses these types of men, is not facing up to the psychological evidence of her life. While no amount of so-called evidence and critical evaluation is a guarantee that one has the "Truth" (because, philosophically speaking, all evidence and facts are discourse-specific and contestable and can never be absolutely adjudicated), nevertheless, what Ecclesiastes is pointing to is the importance of testing one's core convictions about one's life in terms of one's hard-earned experience, and having the courage and good sense to abandon claims that seem to go against the way the world hangs together.

A second attitude towards living that Ecclesiastes articulates and that is fundamental to the psychoanalytic project is that one must learn to live with, that is, accept, what cannot be changed and to submit to that which is impossible to avoid or to prevent from happening (Scott, 1965, p. 205). As Ecclesiastes repeatedly notes, what is cannot be changed by man's efforts, and man does not know, and will never know, why God acts the way He does. In other words, the world keeps moving, regardless of our wishes and our feeble efforts (relatively speaking) to intervene. To understand why time moves in one way and not another is an eternal mystery. Whether we call it providence, fate, luck, or the reality principle, the point is the same—the need to accept life on its own terms because we are not in control of most things, let alone the really important things (e.g., "a time to be born and a time to die": In both instances we have no choice in the matter).

In a similar way, the analysand who was abused and/or neglected as a child, or, for that matter, any patient who has suffered at the hands of his parents or from life's circumstances, needs to be able to accept that that which occurred is a harsh fact of his existence, an event that was out of his control, and, in a certain sense, is an affirmation of the irreversibility of lived time. For after all of the talking, the working through of the personal meaning of the traumatic experiences, finally, the analysand has to accept that what was, was, that it was a *quirk of fate* that he ended up in the circumstances he did (e.g., being born to abusive parents). We know that analysands tend to hold on to their pain and rage since they believe, usually insist, that it should have been otherwise and that they could have (should have) made it different. One way of explaining this is that they do not "fear God", as Ecclesiastes calls it. That is, they are not conscious of His boundless and incomprehensible power (Gordis, 1951, p. 237); they have not fully embraced their helplessness in the context of the arbitrary, capricious, and absolute determinism of life. Without having internalized this notion, that the world and its happenings remain fundamentally unknowable and uncontrollable, one will continue to hold on to one's pain and rage. That man cannot change what was means, in a sense, that he should avoid being fixed in a permanently intense retrospective consciousness, one that is, in part, driven by the angry claim that life is unfair. Moreover, as he does not know what awaits him in the future, good or bad, man should surrender to his fate, that is, it is prudent for him to make the most of the good times while he can, and not be inordinately troubled when things turn bad or nasty (Cohen, 1970, p. 153).

The supreme duty: carpe diem, enjoy life (even if living is a "sorry business")

The logic of Ecclesiastes' philosophy of life could well lead one to conclude that chronic despair is the only option. Given the fragility and impermanence of man's accomplishments, the uncertainty and lack of control of his destiny, the impossibility of his achieving true knowledge, understanding, and insight into the world, and, of course, the inevitability of death, why bother living? However, Ecclesiastes never advocates suicide or despair; rather, he insists that man is Divinely obligated to make joy, including engaging in sensual pleasures, that is, responsible pleasures, the goal of all his activities (Gordis, 1951, p. 252). Says Ecclesiastes,

> Therefore I praise joy, for there is no other good for man under the sun but to eat, drink, and be joyful and have this accompany him in his human toil, during the days of his life, which God has given beneath the sun. [VIII: 15, translated by Gordis, 1951, p. 174]

As Gordis (1951, p. 83) notes, Ecclesiastes

> sets up the attainment of happiness as the goal of human striving, not merely because he loves life, but because he can not have justice and wisdom [i.e., Truth]. Joy is the only purpose that he can find in a monotonous and meaningless world, in which all human values, such as wealth, piety, and ability, are vanity, where all men encounter the same fate and no progress is possible.

In other words, for Ecclesiastes, the only certainty that he has is that man has an intrinsic desire for happiness. Because God created man, He also created this desire; therefore Ecclesiastes claims that God's fundamental purpose for man is the deepening and expansion of his pleasures and the striving after happiness. To fail to obey this Divine commandment is to be a sinner (*ibid.*, p. 115). I would add that it is also foolish. For, as Ecclesiastes eloquently notes, it is the most sensible goal to enjoy life with all the relish one can muster, especially in one's youth, because man is vulnerable to the sudden and often cruel twists of fate, to physical decline, and to death, the end of all activity, which awaits him soon enough.

As in Freudian psychoanalysis, a degree of Stoic fatalism and Epicurean hedonism have their expression in Ecclesiastes' philosophy of life. Putting aside his religious language and categories, his conclusion that the striving after pleasure and joy is a fundamental human motivation and goal is, of course, entirely compatible with the Freudian project. The questions that remain to be answered are what exactly constitutes joy and pleasure for Ecclesiastes, how is it best attained, and what tends to work against experiencing it. It is impossible to detail all of this here, but a hint of what Ecclesiastes has in mind may be helpful.

For Ecclesiastes, like Freud, joy and pleasure are palpable, sensual, and concrete experiences. For example, Ecclesiastes recommends,

> Enjoy life with the woman who you love
> Throughout all the vain days of your life,
> Which God has given you under the sun.
> Throughout your brief days,
> For that is your reward in life
> For your toil under the sun.
>
> Whatever you are able to do, do with all your might, for there is neither action nor thought nor knowledge nor wisdom in the grave towards which you are moving.
> [IX: 7.10, translated by Gordis, 1951, p. 178]

Ecclesiastes is here advocating the importance of a love relationship (of any persuasion) and zestful and purposeful activity to attaining a degree of happiness. No psychoanalyst would disagree with this. However, what Ecclesiastes adds here is rarely emphasized in the psychoanalytic narrative, yet it is an insight that can only heighten the satisfaction associated with love and purposeful activity. I am referring to the fact that the enjoyment of these experiences is enhanced by a greater mindfulness of the transitory nature of life. Moreover, it is this sense of resignation in the face of the brevity of life, in the face of life's all too frequent frustration and harshness, that makes these experiences that much more enjoyable and lasting. Such an attitude also fosters one of the most underrated sensibilities in the modern secular world, a sensibility that religious traditions have emphasized as fundamental to attaining a degree of happiness, a sense of gratitude for what one has. For Ecclesiastes, a certain "downsizing" of one's narcissism is a prerequisite for even episodic and praiseworthy pleasure, let alone a more solid and lasting sense of happiness.

In contrast, Ecclesiastes mocks the masses of men who choose to live their lives in a way that is not mindful of its tragic character. These are the narcissists and, for example, those who are driven by envy and greed, who do not embrace with melancholic resignation (though without despair) the absolute limitations on existence, and who have not cultivated a sense of gratitude for that which they do have. Such people insist that they are masters of their own destiny, that through seeking and attaining more and more acquisitions they will be forever safe and happy.

In other words, in a number of different contexts, Ecclesiastes criticizes as vanity those who fetishize their existence. Fetishization, as I mean it, is "the organization of perception and action, by the personality, around a very striking and compelling—but narrow theme", such as money (Becker, 1969, p. 85). Such a person, says Becker, builds himself firmly into his cultural world, so that he is imprisoned in his own narrow behavioural mould, that is, there is a lack of authentic openness and responsiveness to others and the environment. The reason a person artificially inflates a small domain of the world and over-invests in it, insinuates Ecclesiastes, is that it represents a domain that he can tightly hold on to, can skilfully manipulate, and can use easily to justify himself, his actions, his sense of self, and his options in the world. In psychoanalytic parlance, such a person is neurotic, in that he demonstrates, for example, an extreme conceptual and behavioural poverty, the blocking of the forward momentum of action and the restriction of experience.

Ecclesiastes is particularly hard on those who lust after wealth:

> He who loves money will never have enough of it and he who loves wealth will never attain it—this is indeed vanity. For as wealth increases, so those who would spend it, hence what value is there in the owner's superior ability, except that he has more to look upon? [V: 9–10, translated by Gordis, 1951, p. 158]

Ecclesiastes is here critiquing those who make money or, symbolically, any acquisition their primary focus of self-value, the centre of their universe. Whether it is classical greed, or diligence and thrift, which, for Ecclesiastes, are subspecies of greed, or the quest after fame and power, which he says is frequently rooted in envy and the desire to compete with and outdo others, Ecclesiastes is making an insightful observation that psychoanalysis could benefit from: that the attempt to generate an absolute, closed, narrow, and concrete foundation on which to rigidly base and guide one's existence is seriously misguided. Put somewhat differently, ultimately the realities of life will knock such an arrogant person off his moralistic perch.

Through fetishization, described in Ecclesiastes' terms, the individual denies his creatureliness, he denies God's transcendence and infinitude, and he makes himself the Creator—actually an idolater—as he worships his earthly things. In the psychoanalytic lexicon, such a person is perhaps best described as a malignant narcissist, as one who has developed a primary, self-centred, and driven hedonism that becomes an unhindered and toxic egoism. Such a person forecloses any contact with a source of meaning that remains open, available, and untotalized, whether that meaning is called God or the Other (the latter may be a significant other, says Ecclesiastes—"enjoy life with a woman you love"; Perry, 1993, p. 27). In other words, enjoyment and pleasure from money, fame, power, and sex is ultimately empty and meaningless when it becomes fetishized, that is, becomes a neurotic fixation. However, following Levinas (1985), enjoyment and pleasure can be more. It can be a foundation for individuation, that is, ethical transformation, when it is "sanctioned by the consciousness of the Other" (Perry, 1993, p. 27). To be conscious of the Other, comments Levinas, mainly means to be responsible to, and for, the Other, especially in his suffering (Levinas, 1985, pp. 93–102). As Ecclesiastes cautions us, "Remember your Creator in the days of your youth", that is, when pleasure and joy are most intense and motivating, as in youth, be mindful of the fact—and this is probably even more true in middle and especially old age —that it is the rooting of joy and pleasure in responsibility and care for the Other that is likely to make it the most satisfying, meaningful, and enduring. In other words, the striving after and attainment of money, fame, power, and sex are most likely to be sources of joy, and not sources of malevolent self-transformation, when they are knotted to the ethical relation, when they are first Other-directed and Other-regarding. Moreover, it is the sense of gratitude—in religious language, a consciousness that God has provided one with the means of enjoyment—that encourages the prudent enjoyment of one's acquisitions and pleasures rather than the debasing of oneself or the other by the abuse of them (Cohen, 1970, p. 165).

A final word

I have tried to illustrate some of the brilliant and profound insights about the human condition that are embodied in the ethical wisdom of Ecclesiastes and which may in some form enhance theoretical and clinical psychoanalysis, conceived in this chapter (and this book) as a "practice of the self" (i.e., a method of profound self-transformation and self-mastery). Most importantly, Ecclesiastes advocates resignation without despair, that is, cultivating an inner attitude towards life that strives to transcend the tragic limitations and sorrows of existence through a frank and courageous acceptance that they cannot be transformed. Thus, Ecclesiastes promotes dedicating oneself to striving after joy in life, not so much for the reasons the idealistic pious believe, because it is a gift from God to be treasured, but because the search for joy is the only sensible goal considering the frustrating, tragic, and fundamentally futile nature of existence. Freud probably saw life in a similar way when he famously wrote that purpose of psychoanalysis was to transform "hysterical misery into common unhappiness" (Breuer & Freud, 1895, p. 305).

It is noteworthy that the last six verses of the Book of Ecclesiastes, or so most scholars believe, were written by an orthodox editor who probably was a friend or colleague of Ecclesiastes but who was distressed by his scepticism and perhaps depressive outlook. Although these verses may have been an attempt at damage control, I am convinced that the editor unconsciously wrote verses that capture the very core of what Ecclesiastes believed and advocated, and I believe that they should be regarded as integral and consistent with the rest of the book, at least in my reading of the book of Ecclesiastes: "In sum, having heard everything, fear God and keep His commandments, for that is man's whole duty. For God will bring every deed to judgment, even everything hidden whether it be good or evil" (XIL: 14, translated by Gordis, 1951, p. 190).

Despite all of his uncertainty, ignorance, conflicts, and angst, Ecclesiastes believed that practice—the reality of doing, should not wait for theory, just as life so often docs not wait for understanding and insight (Guthrie & Motyer, 1970, p. 578). What really matters, what perhaps makes life the most meaningful, is the ethical relation, being for the Other before oneself, as Levinas says, and this means, as Ecclesiastes has graciously taught us, creating joy that is rooted and expressed in responsibility to the Other.

CHAPTER FIVE

"Guard your tongue": on the psychological meaning of gossip

> "One who speaks or listens to gossip deserves to be thrown to the dogs"
>
> Rabbi Yisroel Meir Kagan, "The Chofetz Chaim"

In Jewish tradition, and, for that matter, all great world religions (Marcus, 2003), speaking and listening to gossip is regarded as a terrible sin—"God does not accept the prayers of one who speaks gossip," it says in the *Zohar*. (Christianity and Islam, for example, are very hard on those who utter and listen to gossip, rumour, and slander. In the Christian Bible we read, "Being filled with all unrighteousness, fornication, wickedness, covetousness, maliciousness; full of envy, murder, debate, deceit, malignity; whisperers, backbiters, haters of God . . ." [Romans 1: 29–30]. Likewise in Islam, where we read, "Is there anything that topples people on their faces—or he said on their noses into Hellfire other than the jests of their tongues?" [Forty Hadith of An-Nawawi 29]. Quotations from eastern religions that condemn gossip are of a similar nature.) Yet, the fact is that gossip permeates all communities, including the psychoanalytic one. Indeed, as anthropologists and sociologists have noted, gossip has its social significance largely due to its "universality and contemporaneity" (Stewart & Strathern, 2004, p. 200); "One finds gossip to be universal in both time and social space, occurring always and everywhere" (Heilman, 1973, p. 161). Gossip is one of the key modes of communication, underlying people's proclivity for mentally constructing the world they believe in (Stewart & Strathern, 2004, p. 51). In this sense, gossip is also deeply psychological, in that it expresses unconscious wishes, anxieties, needs, and fantasies. Equally important, gossip has a number of important social functions for a community, contributing to the unity, the harmony of opinion, interest, and feeling of a group (Gluckman, 1963), and it allows individuals to seek out their own benefits and self-serving interests within a group context (Paine, 1967). Gossip, sociologically defined, at least in the rudimentary sense, as "information of a more personal nature than rumor; often false, distorted, or blatantly untrue" (Henslin, 1995, p. 695), always occurs behind the gossipee's back and is usually tinged with hostility of some kind. Such easy and unconstrained talk, most often between two people who are friends (or a single "incestuous" group), however, is not always malicious; sometimes gossip is largely positive in intent and consequence, such as when one Freudian analyst tells another Freudian analyst that a colleague who just gave a lecture is "very classical in his approach, psychoanalysis at its best". In this context, the analyst's praise of his colleague is a way of reinforcing the morality of the group, that to be classical in theoretical outlook is a good thing. Moreover, this form of gossip, like most gossip, brings the conversing analysts emotionally closer to each other as they share and affirm their common values and sentiments. Indeed, what can be denoted as "good" or "benign" gossip promotes a feeling of what Alfred Adler called *"gemeinschaftsgefühl"*, that is, a feeling of community.

Gossip, a very slippery concept with no agreed upon definition among researchers (Goodman & Ben-Ze'ev, 1994), is a commanding, influential, and effective social tool that takes many forms and occurs in many different social contexts, each with its situationally specific dynamics, meanings, and interpersonal trajectories. Indeed, what comprises gossip is always context dependent. According to Jaeger, Skleder, Rind, and Rosnow (1994, p. 167), "a piece of information may be gossip in one context, information or news in another, depending on the nature of the social exchange and the intention behind the act". However, in terms of its social significance, gossip, as Stewart and Strathern have pointed out (2004, p. ix), is probably best understood from the point of view of "conflict creation and resolution". Gossip, according to Stewart and Strathern, is always animated by three elements that are extremely important in any group or community, morality, power, and strong emotions (*ibid.*, p. 196). In this essay, I will be focusing largely, though not only, on the individual psychological process involved in gossip, and in the gossiper and the co-gossiper (the listener). Moreover, I will concentrate on what I am calling "bad" or "malignant" gossip, gossip that is meant to be hurtful to the person gossiped about, gossip that consciously and/or unconsciously, directly, or indirectly aims to reduce the status of the other and disrespect his humanity.

Thus, this chapter has three purposes. First, it is an attempt to understand the individual psychology of gossip within its social context—the "fears, resentments, and grievances" (*ibid.*, p. x)—and the anxiety and insecurity that drive, animate, and sustain gossip, a largely psychoanalytically unexplored topic, at least in a systematic way. Second, this chapter aims to suggest that gossip-mongers who engage in malignant gossip, especially habitually, whether analysand or analyst, have unresolved, deep-seated, personal deficits and conflicts that need to be put right. These deficits and conflicts include, for example, truncated ties to empathy, inappropriate ways of expressing aggression and problems with self-esteem maintenance. Most importantly, taken as a constellation of personal limitations, and extrapolating from the path-breaking work of Levinas (Marcus, 2008), the gossip-monger is best understood as being "ethically disabled". As Jacobs (2001) observes, for such people "sound ethical considerations" (p. 1), that is, the for-the-Other of responsibility, are largely "inaccessible to them" (*ibid.*, p. 74). Moreover, such gossip-mongers have a seriously limited capacity for moral self-transformation, "for ethical self-correction". In Levinasian language, a chronic gossiper, like any ethically disabled analysand or analyst, is more or less consistently and significantly estranged from the Good. Such a person is mainly self-centric and selfish, as opposed to other-directed and other-regarding. Finally, I close the chapter with some thoughts about the toxic effects, the social divisiveness, that widespread "bad" gossiping has for the psychoanalytic community.

The collective psychological significance of gossip

Gossip saturates the life of any community; it "has a way of totally consuming one's being and identity" (Heilman, 1973, p. 152). Indeed, in an informal effort to test this claim, I and my wife, also an analyst, found it nearly impossible not to gossip in some form even for as little as half an hour when we socialized with some fellow analysts. As Gluckman correctly noted, "every single day, and for a large part of each day, most of us are engaging in gossiping" in one form or another (1963, p. 308). This being said, as already noted, it is important to be mindful of the fact that there are at least two poles to gossip: a constructive "pole of integration" and positivity in which gossip avoids and resolves conflicts, and a destructive pole of disintegration and negativity in which it generates hostility and disruption. Gossip, in other words, is often an ambiguous social process (Stewart & Strathern, 2004, pp. 202, 30), with diverse intentions and meanings, best conceptualized along a "gossip continuum" (Heilman, 1973, p. 167) from benign to malignant. In this section, I wish to summarize some of the pertinent literature on the collective psychological significance of gossip, which will help to contextualize the main part of this study, which is the individual psychology of gossip, viewed mainly through a Levinasian-inspired psychoanalytic perspective.

Though gossip as a technical term is hard to pin down, for a communication to be regarded as gossip it must satisfy certain minimal requirements (*ibid.*, p. 174): the communicated information must be about the personal life of the target person; it must identify the individual by name or in some other obvious way; it is socially significant only to a particular group of others; and it tends to generate further gossip. So, for example, when an analyst colleague said to me in passing about another colleague of ours, "Between you and me, I don't know why Dr X is regarded as such a 'big shot', all of what he writes about has been said before, and better", he is satisfying the minimum requirements of gossip. Indeed, my felt-as-obligatory response, "Yeah, I know what you mean", which was provoked by my colleague's comment, completed the gossip exchange. My response highlights an important reason why gossip is so summoning for the individual, which is that to be considered part of the group by other members, one needs both to listen to and, to some extent, speak gossip. In other words, to refuse gossip, or to be an excessive non-gossiper, is to refuse "friendship, communion and intimacy" (*ibid.*, p. 166), which, if repeatedly done, is to commit social suicide.

The innovative work of Gluckman (1963) aptly describes some of the positive functions of gossip, which are that it contributes to group unity, cohesiveness, and solidarity. It does this in three basic ways (Stewart & Strathern, 2004, p. 37). First, gossip reinforces and strengthens the morality of a group, the standard pattern of behaviour that is considered "normal" in a particular society. Such norms are supported by the group's maintaining the symbiotic, though dynamically delicate, relationship between the individual's interests and the group's needs, especially in what is considered acceptable behaviour. For example, when a colleague told me that Dr Y undeservedly became a training and control analyst because his best friend, the head of the committee, handpicked the other committee members (he "packed" the committee), with the result that Dr Y easily passed the evaluation, he was reinforcing the idea that only deserving analysts (deserving in his judgement) should be allowed to become training and control analysts. In other words, such a comment was a way of trying to keep others in their place, to keep incompetents and "want-to-bes" out of positions of power (to maintain so-called "standards"), and, thus, to uphold the valued social structure within the institute with its hierarchal division of analysts into training and control analysts ("chiefs"), other analysts ("commoners"), and trainees ("slaves") (*ibid.*, p. 34). Gossip, in this instance, affirms, to the gossiper and to others, their higher status as members and insiders of a group, mainly by a process of self-demarcation, that is, by marking "themselves off from others" by speaking about one another (Gluckman, quoted in Heilman, 1973, p. 158).

Gossip also controls the individual conduct of the group's membership. As Boehm notes (1984), gossip is a sort of "courtroom" (p. 83) in that it "functions as a system through which the group's idea of what should be morally acceptable or unacceptable is continuously rehashed and refreshed" (*ibid.*, p. 84). For example, when one analyst despairingly tells a colleague that the three times a week personal analysis requirement for trainees at institute "N" is not rigorous enough compared to her institute's four times a week requirement, she is asserting her institute's and her own superiority. In addition, in an important, ideologically charged context (Stewart & Strathern, 2004, p. 30), where legitimacy, in part instantiated by personal analysis requirements, is an issue, she is drawing a clear line between those who are inside and outside what she believes is her superior and more legitimate group. In other words, gossip locates a group in relation to other groups and maintains its solidarity as a select, privileged "cream of the crop" group (Heilman, 1973, p. 160).

Gossip is also a potent tool in helping to facilitate choices of leaders by providing a fairly accurate assessment of character and talent in terms of "reputational judgments" that permit the choosing of leaders most likely to do the most good and least amount of damage to the group (Emler, 1994, p. 134). Needless to say, such gossip can destroy reputations, severely compromise relationships, and seriously change the balance of power in an institute, even bring down a respected institute (Ayim, 1994, p. 96). Gossip, as a back channel of information, information not easily available by conventional, official channels (the received discourse), can also be used to obtain knowledge of the political attitudes of new institute leadership or the personal details and circumstances of potential leaders (*ibid.*, p. 95).

Gossip, especially gossip circles (gossip sub-units), can also help control ambitious, power-seeking individuals and make possible the choice of leaders, often without embarrassment, friction, or other types of discomfort (Gluckman, 1963, p. 308). Without embarrassment, because the gossip is done in the "back stage", as Goffman (1961) acutely describes it, the non-public domain, where "we can let our hair down and be ourselves" (Post, 1994, p. 65). For example, in the psychoanalytic community, within the life of an institute where all members are not equal, gossip can be manipulated by the powerful against others, especially the socially weaker. When an incumbent older training analyst running for an institute office mentions in passing to a colleague that his younger non-training analyst opponent once had an affair with one of his previous students, such a betrayal of a "secret" (a special kind of gossip in gossip typology) is meant to diminish his opponent and advance the gossiper's own interests. However, sometimes the less powerful use gossip against the more powerful by causing embarrassment, using such slanderous gossip as, the older "Dr X no longer really practises analysis any more, he is more into giving medication to his patients [a put down among analysts], playing institute politics and retiring. My friend, a neurologist who knows him, thinks he is nearly senile." The gossiper denigrates Dr X in an impossible-to-verify way (a feature of all gossip) by the co-gossiper, and, thus, advances the gossiper's desire to get more referrals of lucrative analytic patients and advance his personal status. That gossip can be used by both the powerful (e.g., to subjugate others) and the less powerful (e.g., as a kind of political resistance), including within the context of choosing leaders, illustrates Gluckman's important observation that "the more exclusive the group, the greater will be the amount of gossip in it" (Gluckman, 1963, p. 309). That is, groups for whom exclusivity and exceptionality is identical with survival tend to generate extreme and recurrent gossipers (Heilman, 1973, p. 162). This is because, in an exclusive group, those who are of high or superior status will try to exert control over others by gossiping with their equals, while those who are lower in rank, status, and importance will try to subvert the power of their superiors by comparable forms of gossip (Stewart & Strathern, 2004, p. 33). Gossip, as Stewart and Strathern point out, which often focuses on the most small-minded matters, "the pettiest details and circumstances" (p. 56), those issues that actually concern people the most in their everyday life, is a vital weapon in "in-fighting" and "back-biting" (*ibid.*, pp. 38–39). In extreme contexts, gossip can lead to rumour ("unsubstantiated information, true or untrue" [*ibid.*, p. 21] that is orally transmitted) and scandal (news that is clearly harmful to those it is aimed against). Whereas gossip and rumour technically need not be harmful, they usually are. In addition, say Stewart and Strathern, rumour may sometimes get into gossip circles, just as scandal may infiltrate both, and, therefore, that which is spoken about becomes more public, potentially more harmful. From gossip, other types of more stigmatizing and degrading social processes directed at the gossipee can also be set in motion, including ugly scapegoating. Gossip, in other words, can "snowball" and become dangerous, even lethal.

Remember, for example, that gossip and rumour were significantly involved in the origins of the Salem witch trials and the Nazi mistreatment of Jews and other minorities.

In summary, following Heilman, we can say that the collectively orientated psychological significance of gossip lies in the support it gives for the group's so-called ego needs, what a group needs to survive and flourish. Gossip is a way of exercising, asserting, and reinforcing communal values and feelings, consolidating and solidifying group identification, sustaining group cohesiveness, and emotionally regulating the group and the individuals that give it its very character and life. Moreover, gossip not only differentiates insiders from outsiders (e.g., Freudian institute "X" from Relational institute "Y"), but can also be used to distinguish various strata of insiders (training–control analysts, regular members, trainees). Thus, gossip may be a means of classifying the group membership, differentiating intra-group cliques (gossip circles, those "in the know", from those who are outsiders), and validating various kinds of relationships from the most fleeting and impersonal to the most long-standing and intimate. In other words, "in its content and patterns of exchange, gossip reflects" (Heilman, 1971, p. 162) what Goffman called "the relational structure of the individual's social world" (*ibid.*, p. 163), that is, how people are interconnected. In this sense, gossip is an extremely important way in which individuals use their "moral imagination" (Stewart & Strathern, 2004, p. 4) to find their way and better "manage" their social world, a world that is often experienced as confusing, anxiety-provoking, and threatening, It is to this subject that we now turn.

The individual psychological significance of gossip

I have emphasized that, in general, gossip, or at least certain forms of gossip, has a positive function in terms of group survival, in particular, as Gluckman has noted, how it defines the boundaries of a community. Gossip, as one researcher indicated, can powerfully inform, strongly influence and thoroughly entertain (Jaeger, Skleder, Rind, & Rosnow, 1994, p. 167).

However, some gossip, especially when it is chronic, can be personally devastating to the gossipee and to the morale of the community. In the scholarly literature on gossip, it is the work of anthropologist Robert Paine (1967) that perhaps most represents a different view from Gluckman's more functionalist outlook. Paine believes that gossip is a type of relaxed, easy "informal communication", and also a mechanism meant to advance, look after, and, if necessary, defend individual interests (p. 278). In this sense, it is also "a catalyst of social process" (Stewart & Strathern, 2004, p. 37). According to Paine, gossip accomplishes its main goal, self-advancement and self-aggrandizement, in two basic ways: it degrades others and it strives to enhance the status of the gossiper at the expense of the gossipee (Paine, 1967).

In this section I want to summarize what I think are the main personal reasons, the motives why people engage in malignant gossip, gossip that is meant to be harmful to the gossipee. While this chapter has not provided a systematic, psychoanalytically informed typology of gossip, a subject worthy of a book, I want to explicate some of the psychosocial dynamics of gossip from the point of view of the three elements mentioned earlier that exist in all intact groups and communities: morality, power, and strong emotions. These three elements loosely correlate with what I believe are the three main deficits that chronic gossipers of the "bad" gossip variety tend to have: truncated ties to empathy (e.g., reduced sympathy and compassion towards others), deficits in self-regulation, that is, in the appropriate expression and management of aggression (e.g., pronounced wishes to dominate, inordinate anger, resentment, jealousy, and envy), and problems in self-esteem maintenance (e.g., an enfeebled self in which there is a lack of confidence in one's own merit as an individual). I will take up each of these deficits as an isolated category, though they are interrelated and interdependent intrapsychic and interpersonal processes. However, before proceeding in my discussion, I want to remind the reader what I mean by malignant gossip in a concrete, real-life sense. Malignant gossip, always treacherous, since it is spoken behind the gossipee's back, manifests itself in, for example, saying something to a co-gossiper that is deliberately hurtful or hostile about a colleague, friend, or family member; circulating a negative rumour about someone else; telling a secret, especially an awkward or embarrassing secret, that a person promised to keep; distorting or lying about something at the gossiper's expense; and "raining on someone else's parade" (like spilling the news that your colleague has been made a training and control analyst before he has let anyone know). Most importantly, in all of these instances, the gossiper, often motivated by meanness, vengeance, or spitefulness, wants the gossipee to be hurt, and that his trust should be compromised and a relationship radically subverted, if not broken up (www.SixWise.com, 2009).

Gossip as truncated ties to empathy

What we take to be acceptable morality, the standards of conduct that are generally viewed as right or proper in our culture, is, to some extent, based on our capacity to empathize with the needs and wishes of others. Empathy, psychoanalytically defined as "the imagining of another's subjective experience through the use of one's own subjective experience" (Person, Cooper, & Gabbard, 2005, p. 551), is a crucial element of our capacity to behave morally, that is, as Levinas says, according to the "for-the-Other" mode of being, to feel responsible for the needs and interests of the Other, often before oneself, and to act accordingly. Clearly, someone who chronically gossips has an insufficiently developed ability to identify with and understand another person's feelings or difficulties, suggesting that the gossiper also has narcissistic problems (a subject we will return to in greater detail in the section of self-esteem maintenance). His failure to honour the reasonable and legitimate needs of the Other not to be harmed are superseded by the gossiper's self-interest. Disrespecting the Other for the sake of self-affirmation and self-aggrandizement is the governing principle of such gossipers and, for that matter, all ethically disabled persons. The claim that malignant gossipers have truncated ties to empathy may at first appear to be stating the obvious. However, there is an important paradox at work here, one that puts the psychoanalytic notion of empathy—"the imagining of another's subjective experience through the use of one's own subjective experience"—into question, or at least in need of ethical deepening. As one "in praise of gossip" scholar noted, "gossip helps us to understand other people in general; by paying attention to details of their lives, we assess evidence for inductive generalizations" (Collins, 1994, p. 112). Collins continues:

> Gossip is a foothold for developing empathy because it discusses particular cases in detail. Gossip also enhances our capacity to project ourselves into increasingly alien circumstances and perspectives, and by evoking uncontrolled and serendipitous details, it enables the imagination to construct unexpected views of its subject. [*ibid.*, p. 113]

Moreover, says Collins, through gossiping, including the knowledge gathering that it involves, we better understand the gossipee's uniqueness and difference, his Otherness, as Levinas would say, and, thus, this questionable argument goes, we develop greater empathy. Finally, by increasing our empathy, we are afforded the opportunity to "check our moral intuitions" and "revise our moral views" of others and sometimes of ourselves (*ibid.*). There is a major flaw in this view of gossip, especially, but not only, regarding malignant gossip, that gossip increases empathy and moral process. This flaw is also pertinent to how analysts generally use the concept of empathy. Empathy, the capacity to put oneself in the other's shoes, is only a positive intrapsychic and interpersonal process when it is attached to, and animated by an other-directed, other-regarding valuative attachment. Empathy that is not mainly for the Other, that is not tied to helping others, altruism, and social responsibility, is often the basis for an act of interpersonal violence, as in the case of malignant gossip.

The main reason that gossip is not positively empathic is that though the gossiper is technically empathizing with the gossipee and co-gossiper, he does so for his own self-serving reasons. While social psychologists have shown that, ideally, say in altruistic behaviour, when the other is conceived as part of the self (i.e., the other's feelings are my feelings, the other's needs are my needs), then helping the other is, therefore, conceived as helping the self. In the case of the gossiper, the empathic process has a different, destructive trajectory. In this scenario, unlike in pro-social empathy, the gossiper does not set what can be called the selfish self aside. Rather, he relates, organizes, and processes all information to himself; his efforts to imagine the world through the gossipee's eyes, his interest in the other, is for his own self-serving ends (Taylor, 1994, pp. 45, 42). Thus, we have what I am calling ethically-guided empathy, empathy that reflects the workings of the ethical self, and exploitative empathy, empathy that reflects the workings of the selfish self. Psychoanalysis at its best, when empathy is focused only on the well-being of the analysand, is an example of ethically-guided empathy, while the empathy that the psychopath uses to deceive and manipulate his victim is an example of exploitative empathy. According to Levinas, empathy that is not mindfully tied to the Good is almost always malicious.

In the case of the gossiper, the central problem, as it relates to his "empathic gap", is that while he is capable of cognitive empathy, the capacity to view things from another person's vantage point, he lacks sufficient affective empathy, the capacity "to experience affect or emotion in response to others' emotional experiences" and to use this experience in the service of a "for-the-Other" moral process (Dovidio & Penner, 2001, p. 183). Without adequate affective empathy, the gossiper is not able to engage in pro-social thoughts, feelings, and, most importantly, actions, such as not to gossip. In this view, gossip reflects the lack of ethically-animated empathy, concern for the well-being of others and social responsibility. By violating the gossipee's right to privacy with utter indifference, by "trivializing" the gossipee's experience, by not adequately considering the negative impact of the gossip on the gossipee's life, the gossiper is acting in an ethically disabled manner. Gossip, in other words, functions as a way of acquiring "illegitimate pleasure" (Taylor, 1994, p. 45) and self-aggrandizement at the expense of the gossipee, especially behind his back, and, thus, represents a stunning failure to recognize another's "dignity and value" (*ibid*. p. 43) as a person.

Gossip as a deficit in the self-regulation of aggression

Examples of gossip's power-seeking and aggressive expression are when it is used as an instrument of social critique or criticism and as a weapon against imagined or real threat, or "perceived domination" (Stewart & Strathern, 2004, p. 58). Indeed, whether it is the "scuttlebutt" in the army, the "poop" provided by the "Stoolie" in the prison, or the "grapevine" (Rosenbaum & Subrin, 1963, p. 818) in the analytic institute, all of us, as social actors, are aware that gossip is potentially dangerous to our well-being, and that it is prudent to keep "one's ear to the ground", as the saying goes.

In order to better understand the gossiper's problem in the self-regulation of aggression, it is important to bear in mind two facts about the social context of gossip. First, historically and typically, gossip (and rumour) takes place within the context of "social malaise, disturbance and anomie" in circumstances that are characterized by high levels of "uncertainty, stress, and perceptions of danger" (Stewart & Strathern, 2004, p. 195). Add to the mix that in certain sites, such as university departments or psychoanalytic institutes, where "hostilities, antipathies, and patterns of opposition" (*ibid.*, p. 201) and self-serving desires may be high, and we can understand why malicious and other gossip may emerge. Second, it is widely believed that people who are particularly anxious and, for example, score high on the Taylor Manifest Anxiety test, tend to spread more gossip and rumours than those who are less anxious (Nevo, Nevo, & Derech-Zehavi, 1994, p. 182).

Gossip, in other words, may be understood as a way of reducing perceived severe threat and anxiety to the self, a way of shoring up and shielding an enfeebled self. Moreover, as a self-protective and self-enhancing expression of power, it allows the discharge of aggression (e.g., anger, envy, revenge), while avoiding dangerous confrontation, open conflict, and additional injury to the self. Thus, through gossiping, the gossiper both repairs and strengthens an inadequately functioning self (e.g., increasing self-esteem and a sense of control), in which gossip acts as an outlet for "letting off steam", usually with minimal risk to himself and to the community. According to this formulation, gossip can be said to have a kind of therapeutic impact on the gossiper's self-concept (*ibid.*).

The main threats that the gossiper may feel to his narcissistic equilibrium, to his sense of worth, competence, and attractiveness, are, of course, varied and depend on the personal history and psychological vulnerabilities of the gossiper. Often they can be traced back to unresolved sibling rivalry (e.g., tattling on a sibling to enhance the relationship with the parent) and Oedipal problems (e.g., when a mother and son gossip about the father, a way of mastering the son's murderous wishes towards the father) (Rosenbaum & Subrin, 1963). Jealousy, envy, and competition, combined with an inordinate need for status (acknowledgement and mirroring, in psychoanalytic parlance), power, and control, are what typically most threaten the gossiper's self-esteem and security. In this context, gossip can provide a temporary antidote to his enfeebled self, as it provides a degree of encouragement, empowerment, and reassurance that the gossiper is not what he thinks and feels he is, which is an endangered "loser".

Finally, and this is crucial, the gossiper has a superego lacuna, an empathic gap in his ability to compassionately consider the gossipee, the "Other", in Levinas's language, before himself, before he satisfies his own inordinate narcissistic needs and desires at the expense of the Other's dignity and value. Put more starkly, whereas the ethically disabled gossiper analysand says, "You [the gossipee] suffer, therefore I am", the Levinasian-inspired, other-regarding analysand says, "I suffer, therefore you are." In other words, in part because of a diminished capacity to experience genuine guilt, the awareness of having done wrong to another accompanied by feelings of regret or shame, the gossiper is not able to generate a more pro-social way of satisfying his neurotic and inordinate narcissistic needs.

Gossip as a form of self-esteem maintenance

It is widely accepted in social psychology literature that low self-esteem individuals are especially motivated to seek approval through impression-management, that is, to try to project favourable, "socially desirable impressions of themselves" (Leary, 2001, p. 459). Presumably, according to Leary, such individuals are highly motivated because "their low self-esteem signals low relational evaluation" (how they think others think about them) (*ibid.*, p. 465). In other words, though all of us are motivated to maintain positive, if not flattering images of ourselves, and to feel good, if not great, about ourselves, the low self-esteem person is inordinately motivated to make good impressions on other people. Thus, the gossiper uses gossip, among other strategies, to maintain and enhance his perceived "relational value to other people" (*ibid.*, p. 471). For the malicious gossiper, the self he knows and the self he shows, his self-esteem and self-presentation, are inordinately driven by his over-determined and exaggerated need to guarantee acceptance by others and to be highly socially valued (*ibid.*, p. 472). Most importantly, the gossiper's excessive efforts at self-enhancement (e.g., satisfying his sense of entitlement, specialness, and privilege within a gossip circle) are always done at the expense of the value and dignity of others, this being an expression of his ethical disablement.

Another important way that gossip enhances self-esteem is through the process of social comparison (Suls & Goodkin, 1994, pp. 174–175). Through the gossip interchange, especially listening to gossip, information is gathered in order to compare oneself to others. These often unconsciously self-servingly distorted comparisons allow for an evaluation of one's own achievements and abilities, and the development of an enhanced self-concept and increased self-esteem. One can, for example, increase one's self-esteem, in particular one's status, by circulating gossip about others, either by attaching or in some way relating oneself to high status individuals or by disparaging them. In addition, by comparing oneself with others worse off, what is called downward comparison, the gossiper can increase his self-esteem. In other words, by circulating negative information about the gossipee, the latter is in an inferior social position compared to the gossiper, which shores up the self-esteem of the gossiper and co-gossiper. Finally, and this is an example of a more benign form of gossip, gossiping about people who are "worse off" provides a chance—a psychological context, to make one's own circumstances appear better to oneself and others, while avoiding real-life interaction or direct contact with those who are less fortunate (*ibid.*, p. 174).

Thus, we can say that the gossiper often suffers from reduced self-worth and self-respect, social anxiety, and an inordinate need for regard, attention, and admiration from others. Malevolent gossip mainly helps to maintain and bolster self-esteem by enhancing the gossiper's sense of status and power; however, this is always achieved by denying the worthiness, respect, and honour of the Other, that is, the gossipee.

A word on gossip in the psychoanalytic "community"

As I have described it, gossip has both a positive and negative significance in the analyst's relationship to the psychoanalytic community. On the positive side, "good" gossip helps analysts better understand the social structure in their training institutes and national and international societies. Gossip helps analysts to function more effectively in their institutes and societies by providing inside information and knowledge about other analysts, their patterns of networking and affiliation, their quirks and individual habits, and location in the hierarchy (Emler, 1994, p. 132).

While a certain amount of relatively benign gossip is inevitable, if not necessary for any community or group to survive and flourish, there is a fine line between when gossip is community-maintaining and community-destroying. Widespread malignant gossip may become dangerous to a community, seriously undermining its integrity and morale. (Incidentally, too little benign gossip is also destructive to a community, in that without such an outlet for tension reduction, an individual may feel overly socially controlled.) For example, the so-called psychoanalytic community, like the academic community, neither of which is, strictly speaking, a community, as is the fellowship of firefighters, but, rather, "a coterie of rival interest-based quasi-groups" (Steward & Strathern, 2004, p. 36), is much more likely to cultivate competitive and hostile, rather than benign, gossip. Thus, too much of the wrong kind of gossip in an institute or society can be seriously divisive, even fatal, as it gradually erodes group cohesion, group norms, and group identity, increasing group pressure (Schoeman, 1994, p. 80). Indeed, the history of psychoanalysis, with all of its schisms, antagonisms, rivalries, and training institute/society skirmishings, have been, and continue to be, saturated with malignant forms of gossip.

Conclusion: gossip as a "triple murder"

Taking my inspiration from Levinas, the main emphasis of this chapter has been to suggest that those individuals who engage in malignant forms of gossip suffer from serious problems in their capacity to affectively empathize and self-regulate their aggression and self-esteem. As a result of having such personal deficits, such gossipers can be characterized as ethically disabled. These individuals are prone to put the satisfaction of their own inordinate narcissistic needs for admiration, status, and power before honouring the dignity and value of others. Malignant gossip, in other words, represents a moral failure in the makeup and behaviour of the gossiper.

Such seriously compromised moral personhood is rooted in the fact that the malignant gossiper can be said to be guilty of a "triple murder", as the greatest rabbinical chronicler of the immorality of gossip, the Chofetz Chaim, suggested in his famous book, *Guard Your Tongue* (1975). Gossip, notes the Chofetz Chaim, "kills three people: the speaker, the listener, and the subject" (p. 183). Unpacking this insight will be a most fitting conclusion to my essay, for it highlights the terrible personal violence that malignant gossip inflicts not only on the gossipee and the co-gossiper, but also on the gossiper. Moreover, such an analysis of gossip puts into sharp focus my broader thesis that psychoanalysis would be greatly enhanced if it developed a moral hermeneutic, especially in the ethical sense that Levinas described, that is more central to its theory and practice.

Words are "loaded pistols", Sartre said in *Qu'est-ce que la littérature?* (1973). Indeed, gossiping can destroy the gossipee's reputation, it can obliterate relationships, and it can cut deeply into a person's self-concept and self-esteem. In a word, malignant gossip, which often grows out of the fertile breeding ground of more benign habitual gossiping, can be soul-murdering to the gossipee. Gossip can also cut deeply into the co-gossiper, in that it can profoundly negatively change how one sees the gossipee. For example, my view of, and way of being with, a respected analytic friend/colleague was forever corrupted when another colleague told me in confidence that my friend had been arrested for shoplifting a few years ago. Such gossip killed something inside me so that I was never again able to be as close to, or honest with, my friend, who never knew that I knew about his arrest. Our trusting relationship had been irrevocably poisoned; my friend was murdered in my eyes by my other friend's malevolent gossip. In addition, my view of my gossiping friend changed, I wondered why he had to tell me what he did. My view of him as a decent and trusted friend had also been seriously eroded.

Finally, as I have said, gossip also in some sense murders the gossiper; over time it warps his outlook and diminishes his social effectiveness. The gossiper uses and hurts others to gain increased status, power, and admiration and, by doing so, he is corrupted, sacrificing his soul in his quest for self-aggrandizement. While I am aware that, in most instances, such malignant gossipers do not feel the least guilty about their gossiping, the fact is that they would if they were operating on a higher level of moral integration. It is the work of analysis to help the gossiping analysand to self-correct by helping him to understand, for instance, the sadism and unresolved sibling rivalry and Oedipal issues that often underlie his malignant gossiping and moral failure. However, the gossiper also may suffer in other ways because of his gossiping. Gossip is a risky business. To gossip effectively one cannot be transparent, that is, the co-gossiper must not sense the gossiper's self-serving motivations; otherwise, the gossiper's own reputation will be diminished in the eyes of the co-gossiper. Moreover, those who are habitual gossipers are often gossiped about in return. Sometimes this backfires: those who live by the sword may die by the sword. Last, the malignant gossiper can suffer in a profoundly practical way, in that his selfish behaviour is perceived as going against the common good. As social psychologists have noted, "altruistic" individuals contribute more to the general good than do "selfish" individuals; they are better appreciated, that is, they are "valued by and receive more benefits from other members of their group" (Dovidio & Penner, 2001, p. 177). As a consequence, they are more likely to survive and flourish. The malignant gossiper, in other words, ultimately murders himself. It is for all these reasons that the Chofetz Chaim wisely railed against the violence of gossip. In a certain sense, for the individual who has achieved a "higher" degree of autonomy and integration, especially in the ethical domain, the idea of gossiping has very little, if any, appeal. Such generous spirits have internalized two ethical principles that they learnt in one of the cultural sites of moral education, the kindergarten: "If you have nothing nice to say, don't say anything at all". The valuative attachments, the lived essence of the Levinasian-inspired, ethically-infused psychoanalysis that has informed and inspired my discussion of gossip, is one that cherishes kindness and silence. As the Chofetz Chaim poignantly quotes from a famous midrash, "For every second that a person remains silent, he will merit reward of a magnitude that is beyond the comprehension of even angels" (Chofetz Chaim, 1975, p. 187).

CHAPTER SIX

The life and soul of good parenting: on wanting, having, and raising children

"Children begin by loving their parents. As they grow older they judge them. Rarely, if ever, do they forgive them"

Oscar Wilde

To be honest, I had always had at least a tinge of envy of Felix, my fifty-two-year-old colleague. He was single, though living with a wonderful forty-year-old woman, nurturing, smart, good-looking, and an accomplished lawyer. The two of them seemed to have a nearly perfect life, a solid relationship, fulfilling careers, and the exciting social and cultural life common to many well-off people living on the upper west side of Manhattan. When I heard from Felix that, even with his stable, bountiful, and satisfying life, he and his partner decided to have a child, I was dumbfounded. Why on earth would they want to upset their enviable lives and have a child, I thought to myself? How could disturbed sleep, dirty nappies, scary illnesses, temper tantrums, and the more or less chronic worry about a child's well-being, be more appealing than their current settled lives?

This chapter attempts to answer this question, to understand what it is about the idea of having a child, "the consummation of erotic life within the structure of the family" (Wyschogrod, 2000, p. 136), that is such a summoning desire. Moreover, why do people like my colleague, and many others with more difficult lives, actually decide to act on their desire to bring a new being into this troubled and troubling world? Finally, and this is the heart of this chapter, once a couple has given birth to a child, how does the parent's self become transformed, how does the self become other through the child, a movement, says Levinas, that accomplishes goodness? Put more simply, in what way does conceiving a child, giving birth to a child, and raising a child, signify, instantiate, and potentiate the ethicality of the parents, the for-the-Other of responsibility?

The conception of having a child

There are many reasons why a couple, especially a loving couple, the focus of this chapter, decides to have a child. These include, for example, a wish to perpetuate themselves, to leave a legacy; if one has a religious sensibility, having a child is a way of doing God's work. From a psychoanalytic point of view, sometimes partners have a child mainly for unhealthy narcissistic reasons, for example, in order to live through their children, or to satisfy some kind of deficit associated with their personal past. The wish to have a child can offer the possibility for a parent to have a corrective emotional experience. As psychoanalyst Selma Fraiberg (1980) noted, the infant is the focal point of transference, with the mother (and father) strongly identifying with the infant and unconsciously evoking a past affective constellation with her own mother, father, or other attachment figure. The intensity of such a reaction is enhanced largely because the infant sets off strong care-giving and nurturing desires as well as compelling contemporary and past attachment emotions (Target, 2006, p. 166). Thus, if the parents are not aware of what is going on in their own minds, child rearing can become a psychologically treacherous ordeal, rather than a joy.

Levinas briefly addressed the issue of why loving partners develop the conception of the child. Why, despite their mutual pleasure and "dual egoism", do partners want to go beyond themselves by having a child (Levinas, 1969, p. 266)? Levinas claims that this movement to have a child goes "beyond the possible" (*ibid.*, p. 281), that "we are before a new category" (*ibid.*, p. 266), a new type of relation, one he calls "fecundity", the capacity to produce a child (Atterton & Calarco, 2005, pp. 45–46). This new "ontological category" (Levinas, 1969, p. 277), along with "paternity", "the way of being other while being oneself" (*ibid.*, p. 282), are conceptualizations that put into sharp focus the ethical basis of the parent–child relationship. In particular, it helps us to understand why a loving couple want to take on the immense responsibility of having and raising a child, and how such a commitment and activity can deepen and widen their ethical subjectivity, their capacity to love, to be for-the-Other before oneself, what Levinas calls goodness.

What Levinas adds to our understanding of why loving couples regard the conception of the child as so summoning is that such a conception points, usually unconsciously, to the possibility of a new mode of being, which is the transcendence of the self in and through an other. Levinas explains this interesting observation:

> I love fully only if the other loves me, not because I need the recognition of the other person, but because my voluptuosity delights in his voluptuosity, and because in this unparalleled conjuncture of identification, in this *transsubstantiation* [roughly, transcendence], the Same and the Other are not united but precisely—beyond every possible project—beyond every meaningful and intelligent power, engender the child. [*ibid.*, p. 266]

The conception of the child "is the possibility" of there being "an other person" (the child) who is in some sense "myself" (the parent), and is also "the reality of myself" (the parent) "in an other" (the child). As Fryer further points out, this "transsubstantiation" permits the self to freely give more "fully to the other" in order to show "responsibility for the other" as not merely "the protection of but also the production of his life" (Fryer, 2004, p. 81). According to Levinas,

> Transcendence—the for the other person—the goodness correlative of the face founds a more profound relation: the goodness of goodness. Fecundity engendering fecundity accomplishes goodness:

> above and beyond the sacrifice that imposes a gift of the owner of giving, the conception of the child. [Levinas, 1969, p. 269]

What Levinas is getting at can be put straightforwardly: the meaning of fecundity, the capacity to produce a child, is that the self is faced with the possibility of a unique relation to the future, a future beyond one's own destiny, a destiny other than one's own, that, nevertheless, at least in some sense, strongly *feels* like one's own. That is, despite the inevitability of old age, illness, and death, one's existence can be prolonged through the production of children (Wyschogrod, 2000, p. 137). Thus, the potential parent in his relation to the imagined child, the idea of the desired child, intuits a way to counteract his unconscious death anxiety. In this unique relation, a way that is both self- and other-affirming, the idea of a child represents a wish to transpose one's self-directed death anxiety to an other-directed responsibility for-the-Other. As we shall see in greater detail, it is mainly because fecundity involves a kind of "doubling and halving of identity", that is, the parent is and is not the child (Llewelyn, 1995, p.130), that the parent feels the summoning responsibility to tend lovingly to his child. Moreover, this anticipated, mainly asymmetrical, intersubjectivity between the parent and the child, a relation in which the parent more or less unconditionally cares for and serves the child as the dependent and vulnerable child grows and develops, actually also includes a crucial element of mutuality. As I noted earlier, the child gives the parent something of infinite worth, something of which George Santayana perceptively observed: "Parents lend children their experience and a vicarious memory; children endow their parents with a vicarious immortality" (Santayana, 1998, p. 104).

The birth of a child

Levinas analyses the effects on parents of the birth of a child as one example of a type of relationship with the Other, theoretically, any Other, which is not merely a relation of knowledge and formal logic, but one of mystery and alterity (otherness). This relation brings about the flight out of being and also implies the dimension of time. He calls such a relation "paternity", though he makes it clear that he is actually referring to an attitude that includes both men and women, fathers and mothers, as they relate to their sons and/or daughters. Levinas's analysis of the birth of a child is mainly concerned with the important issues of what the child represents to the parent, and how such a representation tends to foster the ethical relation. In a word, the child represents possibilities no longer actualizable for the parent, but that are actualizable for the child (Levinas, 1985, pp. 69, 70). Though fecundity/paternity allows the separated self of the parent "to be an other", it is not, paraphrasing Shakespeare, a question of "to be, or not to be, but rather, to be *and* not to be, as the parent both is and is not his child" (Llewelyn, 1995, p. 70). Likewise, as every parent knows, the child, in some sense, is and is not his parent (*ibid.*). That is, his self-identity both resembles his parents in certain ways and is also different from them, uniquely his. Levinas clearly defines paternity:

> The fact of seeing the possibilities of the other as your own possibilities, of being able to escape the closure of your identity and what is bestowed on you, toward something which is not bestowed on you and which nevertheless is yours—this is paternity. This future beyond my own being, this dimension constitutive of time, takes on a concrete content in paternity. [Levinas, 1985, p. 70]

The notion here is that the parent does not simply create his child, but, in some sense, is his child. The parent is considerably and significantly in the child without being the same as the child, "I do not *have* my child; I *am* in some way my child". Moreover, "paternity is not a sympathy through which I can put myself in the son's place. It is through my being, not through sympathy, that I am my son" (Levinas, 1987, p. 91). In other words, paternity is not simply identifying with the child; the alterity of the child is not mainly that of an alter ego. Rather, it is "a relationship of the ego with a myself", who is at the same time "a stranger to me" (*ibid.*).

A useful way of thinking about Levinas's intriguing observation that in parenthood the I both is, and is not, its child is to conceive of the child, that is, raising a child, as a "project in life" (Atterton & Calarco, 2005, p. 47). For example, a "good enough" parent tries to teach his child how to achieve autonomous selfhood. Indeed, as someone once said, perhaps the most crucial thing that parents can teach their children is how to manage their lives, how to survive, if not flourish, without them. Such autonomous selfhood is mainly accomplished through gently conveying to the child what to do, and what not to do, in his life (based mainly on the parent's successes and mistakes made in his own life), while also encouraging him to push himself to venture out into life confidently and hopefully, courageously dealing with life's inevitable disappointments and adversity. In other words, the goal for the parent is to help the child make his own reasonable decisions in life, with the parent being a guiding and helpful influence, without being perceived by the child as too controlling or in other ways undermining. As every good parent knows, such a delicate balance requires great skilfulness, walking the narrow ridge between encouraging the child's freedom and experimentation on one hand, and imposing reasonable limits that engender self-restraint on the other. Within this context, paradoxically, the parent creates the conditions of possibility for the child to create his "own possibilities" (*ibid.*). In other words, the child, to some extent, depends on his parents' transmitted wisdom, the totality of experiences and derived knowledge that constituted his child-rearing, to become autonomous. To the extent that the parents are capable of educating the child to become autonomous, it can be claimed that the parents actualize "one of their possibilities". As Atterton and Calarco further note, "They make possible the possibilities of the child—possibilities that are both theirs (they made them possible) and not theirs (they are possibilities of their child, who is an independent being)" (*ibid.*).

It is worth noting that it is through paternity, a way of being Other while being oneself, that Levinas puts into sharp focus a mode of being that has applicability beyond one's offspring, to all forms of love. In every authentic love relation, on some level, there is an abiding wish to create the conditions of possibility for the Other to create his own possibilities, especially to enhance the Other. In other words, as with one's own significant other, I try to provide him with the space and resources to make good decisions in his life, enhancing the conditions of possibility without attempting to control his deliberations or make his decisions for him, to realize his own possibilities as he views them. This is paternal attitude at its best: I am in his world and yet not of his world, I am, says Stanislas Breton, "inside and outside at once", a condition aptly described by him as the relation of "being towards" (2004, pp. 128, 136).

For Levinas, the relation with the child puts the parent into relation with a new structure of time, what he calls "infinite time". "The relation with the child—that is, the relation with the other that is not a power, but fecundity—establishes relationship with the absolute future, or infinite time" (Levinas, 1969, p. 268). Fecundity, says Levinas, "opens up an infinite and discontinuous time", it is the discontinuity and multiplicity that must be emphasized (*ibid.*, pp. 201, 282).

Infinite time "is the time in which the I exists without the finite limits of mortality" (Atterton & Calarco, 2005, p. 48). "The time in which being and infinitum is produced goes beyond the possible" (Levinas, 1969, p. 281). Infinite time, in a certain sense, is the possibility of a kind of everlasting youth, of newness, of eternal spring and hopefulness; it frees, or nearly frees, the self from the past in that one's mistakes, one's guilt-inducing omissions and commissions, take on new, more life-affirming meaning and purpose (Atterton & Calarco, 2005, p. 48). I am reminded of a convicted felon I interviewed in a maximum-security prison who wanted court-ordered visitation with his four-year-old daughter, whom he had seen only once or twice before he was incarcerated. He told me, "The only thing that makes me want to survive in this jungle is the thought of reunion with 'my baby'. I am finished with a life of crime, all I want is to get out of this hell hole and be a good father to her, to let her know I did not forget her."

Infinite time also frees us from, or at least lessens the frightening awareness of, growing old, becoming sick, and dying. Our good works, such as the goodness that we foster in our children, manifested in their living their lives in a manner that makes the world a better and more beautiful place, means, in a certain sense, that we live on. Fecundity thus brings about goodness in that it is through our children that we transmit important memories and insights and inculcate responsibilities to those who come after us (Hutchens, 2004, p. 87). Levinas calls this release from the past or, at least, the easing of the burdens of the past and release from the mainly egological interiority that fecundity brings about, "pardon" (Levinas, 1969, p. 283).

Pardon is the recurrent "repetition of new beginnings" (Wyschogrod, 2000, p. 137). Beyond all expectations and horizons the parent's future now contains "a new birth of the Other", experienced, perhaps, as "one's own being for the infinite" (*ibid.*). In some sense, through pardon, the parent's past has been liberated from its burden of the irreversibility of lived time. Thus, it is through the birth of the child, says Levinas, that the parent's past time can find a kind of salvation: having a child creates the context for the parent's radical self-transformation and self-transcendence, a sort of glimpse of redemption, this being the child's "gift" to his parents. However, for the newborn child to be the occasion of the parent's unburdening himself of his mistakes in the past, a sort of "second chance", the parent must embrace with the fullness of his whole being his responsibilities for the Other, he must properly take care of and serve the child. In other words, the mystery and magic of fecundity is the way in which it is able to liberate the potential parent's future from inordinate self-centredness and selfishness. It can transform the egoity of the copulating, child-conceiving lovers into the other-regarding ethical subjectivity of parents. It is this transformation of the parent's inner world and outward actions from being mainly for oneself to being for the Other, including understanding some of the difficulties and complexities that this entails in terms of everyday "hands-on" parenting, that we now turn.

Raising a child

Levinas, being the severely abstract and abstruse philosopher he was, did not have much to say about the everyday struggles of real parents raising real children in the real world. However, his abstract insights into the parent–child relationship have direct bearing on one of the main themes of this chapter, which is the way a parent's subjectivity is made more ethical, in the Levinasian sense, as he or she raises their child. In other words, how does this shift "from self-preoccupation to the preoccupation for the responsibility of the Other" (Hatley, 2006, p. 84) play out in the hustle and bustle of everyday life between parents and children?

For Levinas, there are two figures in the real world who perhaps best depict the inner attitude and outer behaviour of persons capable of being good parents, that is, as living their love as responsibility for the Other. The first, the devoted mother, or care-giver, Levinas describes in his discussions of maternity. The second, the master teacher, he only makes passing reference to. I want to describe briefly how the ideal mother and master teacher manifest the form of Levinasian love that I am suggesting constitutes the most important elements of the good parent.

For Levinas, "maternity in the complete being 'for the other' which characterizes it, which is the very signifyingness of signification, is the ultimate sense of this vulnerability" (Levinas, 1998a, p. 108). Alphonso Lingis, in his translator's introduction to Levinas's *Otherwise Than Being* (1998b), says:

> Concretely the acts by which one recognizes the other are acts of exposing, giving, of one's very substance to another. Responsibility is enacted not only in offering one's properties or one's possessions to the other, but in giving one's own substance for the other. The figure of maternity is an authentic figure of responsibility. [*ibid.*, p. xix]

Writing in one of his Talmudic commentaries, Levinas develops one of the core aspects of maternity, the quality I want to focus on:

> *Rakhamim* (Mercy), which the Aramaic term *Rakhmana* evokes, goes back to the word *Rekhem*, which means uterus. *Rakhamim* is the relation of the uterus to the *other*, whose gestation takes place within it. *Rakhamim* is maternity itself. God as merciful is God defined by maternity. . . . Perhaps maternity is sensitivity itself . . . [Levinas, 1990b, p. 193]

In other words, the existential stance that best exemplifies one's responsibility for the other, the essence of good parenting, is one that is characterized by mercy or, in less religious language, compassion. Compassion is a notion that is grossly under-explored in the psychoanalytic literature. Moreover, it is hardly ever a term that analysts use in describing a successful analysis. Meissner, for example, a Jesuit priest–analyst, in his recent book on the ethical dimension of psychoanalysis (2003), does not even list compassion in his index, and Wallwork, in his review article on "Ethics in psychoanalysis" (2005), also does not discuss compassion as part of the deep ethical theory informing the practice of psychoanalysis. In contrast, compassion, sometimes called mercy or loving kindness (e.g., as in Buddhism) is a core virtue of all major wisdom religions of the world (Marcus, 2003).

Compassion, defined straightforwardly as sympathy for the suffering of the other, including a desire to help, especially as manifested in the ideal mother, can be viewed as having at least two dimensions. First, compassion involves the ceaseless, abundant unconditional love for the other. Second, it expresses a love devoted to helping and to steering the other in a new direction. This requires abiding patience, empathy, understanding, and forgiveness. These two dimensions of compassion constitute the engaged love that Levinas seems to be pointing to in his notion of responsibility for the other. Parent–child love, as well as adult love relations, is based on a fundamental obligation to make ourselves fully available, with boundless compassion, to the neediness (in the non-neurotic sense), the suffering, of the beloved child and or significant Other.

Indeed, the child as Other is "the persecutor who teaches me" (Hatley, 2006, p. 83). Persecution, Levinas's evocative term for his claim that I am first and foremost hostage of the Other, that I am persecuted because I cannot escape the priority of the other over me in terms of my responsibility (*ibid.*), is the way in which many parents often actually experience their relationship, their obligations, to their child. Like moral life, according to Levinas, parenthood itself is persecution. In other words, the child as Other, the one who persecutes me in his demands to be continuously cared for and served before myself, is the one who teaches the parent the significance of his responsibility. Put more strongly, the child as persecutor teaches the parent what sacrifice is all about. Sacrifice, a giving up of something valuable or important to oneself for somebody else considered to be of more value or importance, is what mainly constitutes being a good parent. Sacrifice, in other words, is an expression of what Toni Morrison, in her masterpiece *Beloved*, called "thick love", a parent's deep and abiding readiness to do everything required for the sake of her child's best interests. This is not nearly as easy, or as obvious, as it may sound, for as every parent knows, there are many times throughout child-rearing when parenthood seems, as someone once said, nothing but feeding the mouth that bites you. In other instances, a parent's willingness to sacrifice for his child can be a barely disguised form of manipulation and hostility. Think of the stereotype of the Jewish or Italian mother who makes her son feel guilty for all she has done for him. And, finally, too much sacrifice, too much selfless giving can be deleterious to the child, in that his autonomy is not encouraged (e.g., the parent does for the child what he should be encouraged to do for himself). Moreover, as W. B. Yeats wrote in "Easter 1916", "Too long a sacrifice / Can make a stone of the heart". Parents, in other words, can become burnt out from too much sacrifice, a kind of sacrifice overload, especially when the child appears ungrateful and the results of the sacrifice do not lead to a good outcome. This is the moment when a parent experiences his child as persecution in the negative sense. I am thinking of a parent patient of mine whose adult son was a drug addict from age ten, and after years of looking after him and trying to get him the help he needed, after an unbelievable outpouring over many years of emotional, financial, and other forms of sacrifice, she begrudgingly pulled away from him, and told me, "I just don't have anything more inside to give him. It kills me to say this." That this devoted mother could say, "It kills me to say this" speaks to the trace of the sacrificial self as it gives way, wisely, though very sadly, to the pragmatics of maintaining the integrity of her own selfhood, accepting the reality that there is nothing more to be done, and ultimately helping the drug addict by refusing to continue being an "enabler". In many instances, such pulling away from a substance abuser, and letting him hit "rock bottom", as they say in Alcoholics Anonymous, is a necessary precondition for the substance abuser to embrace the necessary self-responsibility and decision-making that are required for recovery.

Forgiveness is the second term I want to mention as a characteristic of the "good enough mother", the responsible subjectivity that is equated with the capacity to love, as Levinas construes it. For the secularist, including the secular psychoanalyst, the word forgiveness, like compassion, is often saturated with religious connotations and meanings, and, therefore, is generally not a crucial part of the dialogue between the typical secular analyst and analysand, nor is it usually part of scholarly psychoanalytic discourse.

Like compassion, forgiveness, the act of pardoning somebody for a mistake or wrongdoing, requires a profound psychological capacity, as well as considerable autonomy, integration, and self-esteem. Not only is the capacity to forgive a prerequisite for being a "good enough", responsible mother or care-giver, it is also necessary for maintaining the integrity and continuity of any love relation.

Levinas seems to be implying the same insight when he boldly and provocatively claims that one is responsible for the persecutor, including one's own, by embracing the responsibilities of the persecutor that are not discerned and manifested (Hutchens, 2004, pp. 24–25):

> In maternity what signifies is a responsibility for others, to the point of substitution for others and suffering both from the effect of persecution and from the persecuting itself in which the persecutor sinks. Maternity, which is bearing par excellence, bears even responsibility for the persecuting by the persecutor. [Levinas, 1998b, p. 75]

In other words, for example, when my child says something offensive and unkind to me (when he persecutes me), it is my responsibility to help him see how he has pained me, and to help steer him back on track. It is my responsibility to demand justice from him, and, in so doing, I encourage him towards greater critical self-reflection, sensitivity, and compassion. Moreover, by pointing out his culpability, I mobilize greater responsibility for himself, in terms of self-control, remorse, and making reparations. This kind of parenting intervention requires great skilfulness, but it is essential for bringing up a child with a sense of personal responsibility, consequential thinking, and empathy.

Forgiveness, a core aspect of responsibility for the other, can foster positive changes in one's emotional life and is an important component to good parenting: it can reduce one's anger, resentment, and retaliatory wishes toward the child; it can renew a parent's sense of self-efficacy, control, and power in that it leads towards a more active and compassionate role in changing how one views one's sense of being mistreated or having mistreated; and, of course, forgiveness can lead to reconciliation between the parent and the child (this dynamic plays out in a big way with teenagers). By forgiving, parents enlarge their options, autonomy, and freedom to grow, develop, and flourish. Forgiveness also encourages children to take responsibility for their wrongdoing, which makes it easier for the offended parent to reduce his hurt and begin the healing process (Richard, Richards, & Bergin, 1997, p. 212). Finally, perhaps, forgiveness also includes transforming one's rage, resentment, and animosity into more constructive and positive sentiments. By forgiving a child who has mistreated you, you, in effect, give up the right to strike back at the child, this being one of the main reasons it is so hard to forgive. While the strong negative emotions associated with the frustration and difficulties of parenting are not usually focused on by those thinking of having children, or even parents who have children, the mindfulness and reasonable "management" of these feelings has an enormous impact on the development of a child, including his moral life. Indeed, through the challenges that the child embodies for the parent in terms of self-mastery, the good parent is "forced" to face himself, sometimes with brutal critical honesty, which often leads to an appropriate sense of guilt for messing things up for the child. Simone de Beauvoir beautifully captured the painfully ambiguous quality of parental responsibility when she wrote, "it is frightening to think that you mark your children merely by being yourself. It seems unfair. You can't assume the responsibility for everything you do—or don't do" (http://www.famous-quotes.com/author.php?aid=571). The child, in other words, widens and deepens the parent's moral life, both by making him critically evaluate where he has gone wrong. According to Oliver Wendell Holmes, "Pretty much all the honest truth-telling there is in the world is done by children" (http://theparentsite.com/parenting/quotes.asp), and then, one hopes, in part out of genuine guilt, the parent tries to put things right. There is an episodic, uniquely disruptive upsurge of guilt and responsibility, and the wish to make reparations, in the parenting experience at its best. I comment further on this very important guilt–responsibility–reparation progression at the end of this chapter.

The second real-life figure who best expresses the key qualities of good parenting, parenting conceived as love as responsibility for the Other, is the master teacher (Levinas, 1996a, p. 21). As Levinas points out, the Other is one's teacher: "The other is . . . the first rational teaching, the condition of all teaching" (Levinas, 1969, p. 203). Moreover, for Levinas the teacher–student relationship initiates the messianic in that the teacher redeems and comforts the student, and points him in the direction of living a life of peace, justice, and compassion.

Being a master teacher involves bringing all of oneself to the student (i.e., the loved other), as opposed to partially attending to the student's words. It involves taking great care of what is given to him. It demands that one be willing and able to do all he can in order to find the best solution to the problem of the student, to ease that which troubles him. In the parent-to-child love relation this includes the everyday "hands on" problems in living associated with school, peer relations, career decisions, and the like.

Responsibility towards one's student also involves attempting, with great gentleness and care, and within the context of profound trust, to disrupt the student, to undermine the security-maintaining walls around him that constitute his taken-for-granted assumptions about himself and the world. The purpose of such disruption is to create the conditions of possibility for the student to think differently. This means encouraging him to create the space inside himself to imagine a wider horizon and, if he chooses, to expand, deepen, and change his perspective on a particular issue and/or to shift his perspective on life. In an educational context, this can be accomplished by the teacher's listening to the student with the fullness of his whole being and responding with the maximum of his intellectual and emotional resources.

The application of this existential orientation of the master teacher to his student is easily recast to the parent-to-child love relation and, for that matter, to most forms of love. In the parent–child love relation, genuine responsibility means helping the child to actualize his human potential. For both a teacher and parent this means acting like a midwife to the soul, facilitating the birth of a new self, a better self, a self capable of growing intellectually, emotionally and morally, and having an increasing capacity for love, compassion, and forgiveness.

The challenge of good parenting

While I have claimed, following Levinas, that a good parent is best exemplified in the ideal mother, conceived as the authentic figure of responsibility and sacrifice, and the master teacher, conceived as midwife to the birth of the child's self, there remains at least one important question, the original question, that Levinas does not adequately answer, at least on the level of real-life parent–child interaction, but which is basic to parenting:

> How, in the alterity of a you, [the child], can I [the parent], remain I, without being absorbed or losing myself in that you? How can the ego that I am remain myself in a you, without being nonetheless the ego that I am in my present, that is to say, an ego that inevitably returns to itself? How can the ego become other to itself. [Levinas, 1987, p. 91]

As we have seen, Levinas is raising key questions, questions that lead him into his description of fecundity and paternity, concepts we have already discussed. However, what he does not adequately describe and explain, or at least give a good sense of, is how all of this actually plays out between the parents and the child within the context of actual social interaction. Without knowing this, in psychoanalytic terms, the intersubjective dynamics, it is extremely difficult to know how best to relate to one's child, how to parent a child so that he or she is more likely to be an autonomous and integrated person, capable of deep and wide love and creative and productive work. Moreover, it is precisely this parental capacity, "to be and not to be" (the parent is and is not his child) that both expresses the unique aspect of the parent's moral life, and, at the same time, assists the child in becoming both who he is and who he wants to be. That being said, to do all of this parental relating mindfully, skilfully, and gracefully, always in the service of the child's best interests, requires a considerably nuanced understanding of, and responsible responsivity to, the self–other interplay.

To understand how, in the alterity of a child, I, the parent, can remain I, without being absorbed or losing myself in that child, we need to describe one of the essential characteristics of the good parent, at least from a Levinasian-inspired, ethically-infused psychoanalytic point of view. The parent needs both to love the child as she loves herself, that is, with the same or similar degree of positive self-concern, self-interest, and self-regard, while also relating to the child as a unique, separate, and individuating other. In other words, to the extent that the parent can generate the cluster of positive feelings, thoughts, and fantasies that are usually focused on oneself, self-involvement on the way to self-enhancement, and direct them towards the child, while simultaneously relating to the child as an independent, developing other, both the child and parent are most likely to flourish, especially morally. In psychoanalytic terms, because children are the result of the intimate synthesis of "physical and personal identities" of the parents, the parents have a strong "libidinal investment" in, and emotional connection to, their children (Monte, 1980, p. 257). Roughly speaking, this is what Levinas is pointing to when he says that the parent is the child. However, as Erik Erikson described in his notion of "generativity", the deep care that the so-called mature adult has with what is generated, children, ideas, and products (Hall & Lindzey, 1978, p. 98), the parent has the capacity to go beyond immediate self-directed interests in favour of a view of the Other (Monte, 1980, p. 257). He can facilitate the best interests of the child and, by extension, the generations of children that follow. Erikson, sounding Levinasian, further notes that the "ego strength" or virtue, as he calls it, that the generative adult develops through such good parenting is that of "care": "*Care is the widening concern for what has been generated by love, necessity, or accident; it overcomes the ambivalence adhering to irreversible obligation*" (Erikson, 1964, p. 131; original italics; Monte, 1980, p. 257). It is through parenting, but also teaching, healing, and other such activities in which the adult acts as the conveyor of the best of social values (Hall & Lindzey, 1978, p. 99), as well as of life-conduction wisdom, that the child's character development, including his moral life, but especially his capacity to give and receive love, develops and thrives. At the same time, the parent's inner world, his sense of the meaningfulness of his own life beyond his physical duration, is enlarged and deepened through his ability to extend himself, to give himself to the future through his role as parent. As we have said, "beyond the possible" is what Levinas calls this parenting ability. Needless to say, says Erikson, those parents who are not able to establish a sense of generativity tend to lose ground, experiencing a pervasive sense of weariness and dissatisfaction, which has a inevitably deleterious effect on their children. In Levinasian terms, such parents are fundamentally impoverished because, unless they have major felt benefits to their own diffuse and inadequately developed sense of self, unless they consistently derive enhanced self-esteem, unless they feel "fed" by their child, a toxic role reversal takes place. The fact of being needed by the child, of being seen as an important person who "knows what they are talking about", is not enough for such narcissistically compromised parents. Such a form of distorted parent–child interaction, with its harmful effects on children, seems to be fairly pervasive these days. As one university-based study of narcissism among American university students, the so-called "Generation Y", has found, there was a 30% increase over 25 years in the number of young Americans with symptoms of "elevated narcissism", with more of them than ever agreeing with such statements as, "I like to be the center of attention", and "I think I am special" (*The Week*, 2007a, p. 19). Indeed, some social scientists have claimed that members of Generation Y seem to be especially preoccupied with themselves, an observation that strikes me as plausible from my clinical experience.

How, then, does the parent's moral relation to the Other, the child, increase the parent's ethical possibilities? In more straightforward psychological language, what are some of the implicit and desirable explicit ethical processes at work between parents and children? In order to answer this question, I will focus on two key aspects of parenting that have great ethical weight from a Levinasian point of view, themes that I have already touched upon but need to further elaborate: empathy and guilt. (I have generously drawn from the thoughtful work of Sharon Todd [2003] in my discussion of empathy and guilt.) As these are large and complex topics in both the Levinasian and psychoanalytic literatures, I will limit my brief concluding comments about these subjects to their relation to the main theme of this essay: how is the parent's self transformed, how does the self become other through raising a child, a movement, claims Levinas, that accomplishes goodness?

Empathy

Unquestionably, good parenting requires a deep and pervasive capacity for accurate empathy, the ability to identify with and understand the child's feelings and difficulties. However, from a Levinasian point of view, empathy is not simply "putting yourself in another's shoes". Rather, as psychoanalyst Elisabeth Young-Bruehl points out, the process of empathy requires being in, but not of, the child, a complex and demanding psychological process, difficult to "pull off" gracefully:

> empathizing involves, rather, putting another in *yourself*, becoming another person's habitat as it were [the child is the parent, says

> Levinas], but without dissolving the person, without digesting the person [the child is not the parent]. You are mentally pregnant, not with a potential life but with a person, indeed, a whole life—a person with her history. So the subject lives on in you, and you can, as it were, hear her in this intimacy. But this, as I said, depends upon your ability to tell the difference between the subject and yourself, which means to appreciate the role that she plays in your psychic life. [Young-Bruehl, 1988, p. 22, quoted in Todd, 2003, p. 203]

Thus, we can say that empathy, at least as I am using the term, involves both being able to put your self inside the other without losing yourself, while, at the same time, being able to put the other in your self without eradicating the other's difference and otherness. Exactly how a self's ego becomes supple enough to incorporate or, more aptly, to bring the other within its experience without necessarily having to project anything upon or into the other, is neither clear nor agreed upon by most psychoanalytic and social psychological theoreticians on empathy.

In terms of the parent's developing ethical potential *qua* parent, what is important here is that empathy seems to be the precondition, the mode of relation, for the parent to parent his child responsibly. In other words, only when the parent responds empathically to the demands of the vulnerable and dependent child through respect and the affirmation of her uniqueness and otherness can the parent generate the kind of togetherness that goes beyond "being-with" the child, to "being-for" the child (Todd, 2003, pp. 46–49). This kind of parental empathic immersion, one that is both within and beyond the child, rooted, in part, in the parent's conscious and unconscious wishes to nurture, protect, and promote the child's well-being, is an act of responsibility that emanates from the special kind of communicative, affectively-infused interchange that constitutes the parent–child relationship at its best. From a Levinasian point of view, what is ethical about empathy is that it demands that the parent not reduce the experience of the child to the parent's self; it requires that the parent let the child reveal herself, in all of her mystery, without the parent trying to eradicate the difference between them (Todd, 2003, p. 51). "The alterity of the Other is in him and is not relative to me; it reveals itself" (Levinas, 1969, p. 121; Todd, 2003, p. 51). Most importantly, perhaps, for the parent to engage the child's otherness in all of its uniqueness and unknowable mystery means to be for her, or rather better put, to be for her first. That is, the parent's overall orientation, his way of listening and responding to the child, needs to be considerably less self-directed and self-interested, and more other-directed and other-regarding. For many parents, this mode of relation comes more or less spontaneously, a kind of emotional openness and susceptibility, possibly hard-wired to some extent, that allows the parent to be deeply "affected", "moved", or "touched" by their child, and to want wholeheartedly to give himself to her (Todd, 2003, p. 53). However, while such non-intentional responsiveness may be the affective bedrock of good parenting, to be properly empathic over the long haul of parenting requires that the parent be mindfully open, receptive, and responsive to the child's otherness, to what makes her unique, and to learn from her. It is precisely this "ethical attentiveness to difference qua difference" that is crucial to empathy, and thus to good parenting (*ibid.*, p. 63). To embrace such a mindful empathic stance is itself an expression of ethical responsibility for the Other, since it moves against the human tendency to be self-interested, and, in our current context, to reduce the Other to some common ground with oneself. Empathy, in other words, creates ethical responsibility and commitment for the parent: in Levinasian terms, goodness through a connection with the child that respects and affirms her unknowable, impossible-to-pin-down uniqueness and otherness.

Guilt

In over twenty years of consulting with parents as a psychotherapist, and being a parent myself, I have yet to meet a parent that did not feel at least somewhat guilty about how he or she has mistreated their child. Whether through acts of omission or commission, whether intentionally (yes, good parents can be mean to their children sometimes) or unintentionally, the fact is that guilt, an awareness of having done wrong accompanied by feelings of regret or shame, is a common sentiment among parents who are honest and thoughtful in their judgement of themselves. For some parents, this feeling is a pervasive sense of wrongdoing, whereas with others it is episodic. As I will suggest, such manifestations of guilt often have their origins and motivational power in a seriously lapsed responsibility for the Other, an experience that has tremendous ethical potential for the parent. This form of guilt, what I am calling genuine or real guilt, is different from the neurotic guilt that psychoanalysis is mainly concerned with. Briefly, a neurotic sense of guilt results from those internal experiences that are not adequately accountable for in terms of violating the individual's consciously held values and moral principles. For Freud, the neurotic sense of guilt emanates from an unconscious, intrapsychic conflict between the superego and the id, the latter standing for those infantile aggressive and sexual wishes that are the touchstones of clinical psychoanalysis.

For Levinas, such genuine guilt reflects the awareness that one has, in a crucial way, let down, if not radically abandoned or betrayed, the other person. To the Other's summoning me to responsibility, despite myself, as Levinas would argue, I have failed adequately to respond with empathy and care to the needy other's call. Most important, perhaps, by ignoring or rejecting the other's plea to be responsible, to give help, I feel that my right to exist is profoundly questioned. Such genuine guilt, insinuates Levinas, can become the awful and inescapable feeling, though ultimately life-affirming "obsession", that inevitably compels me to turn towards the other person with a seemingly impossible to satisfy guilt (Hutchens, 2004, p. 90). Real guilt, says Martin Buber, demands "reconciliation"; it demands making what, in another context and with a somewhat different emphasis, Melanie Klein famously calls reparation: to make good that which one has injured, though it is almost always made worse by conscious and unconscious fantasy. Psychoanalytically speaking, we can, thus, say that neurotic guilt is, in part, a bribe to the superego to avoid the more painful, humiliating, irrepressible, and debilitating experience of genuine guilt. Stated somewhat differently, not confronted, unanalysed genuine guilt can morph into neurotic guilt (May, 1958, p. 55). As is well known to analysts, such avoidance of honest self-confrontation can have far-reaching negative, if not dire, consequences for the self-accused perpetrator of the guilt-worthy action.

For Levinas, then, there is an unqualified demand that arises from the radical otherness of the other, in our current context, the child, a demand that emanates from the direct experience of the child's vulnerability and neediness. Levinas's notion of what we are calling genuine guilt is, in his words, an "accusation", an assumed debt without any choice, one that can never be fully satisfied. For Levinas, guilt is a fundamental, if not formative, aspect of subjectivity. Guilt comes about mainly because one is, from the outset, susceptible and vulnerable, responsive to the other's presence, to the summoning call of the self–other relation itself (Todd, 2003, p. 99). In this sense, then, guilt, or rather genuine guilt, is best viewed as a kind of moral compass pointing us in an other-orientated, other-regarding direction. "The self is bound to the Other in a relation of guilt in which the self bears the burden of the Other's subjectivity, the Other's freedom, and the Other's mortality" (*ibid.*, p. 109). For Levinas, we are guilty because we are susceptible to the Other, the child's presence touches and moves us. We sense, if not feel, utterly accused: the child's anguish causes me anguish. Most important, guilty self-awareness and self-comprehension, the embracing of genuine guilt, always points to action-guiding responsibility (that is what distinguishes it from neurotic guilt). Guilt is a responsible response towards the Other's pain, a response that generates pain for the person who cannot help but feel guilty (*ibid.*, pp. 113, 114).

The application of this Levinasian-inspired analysis of guilt has direct bearing on the parent–child relation. As most parents will tell you, it is their child, in her neediness and vulnerability, whom they experience as the most summoning relationship, especially in the early years of development when the child is literally helpless, exposed, and suffering (e.g., crying, hurting). Parents, in other words, suffer when their children suffer; as the saying goes, a parent is only as happy as his most unhappy child. The point I am making is that a good parent or "good enough" parent is one who is mindful of how they have failed their child (also how they have succeeded so as to keep doing so), a failure that is inevitable, while they try to put things right. This point may sound obvious, but it is an aspect of the parent's developing moral life, embracing with the fullness of his being the guilt–responsibility–reparation mode of relationality, as he mindfully raises his child, which is often downplayed or overlooked. Nietzsche, writing in another context, pointed to the difficulty of such a for-the-Other sensibility when he wrote, "to take upon oneself not punishment, but guilt—that alone would be godlike". Every parent, in other words, is guilty of all the good he did not do for his child, and it is precisely the mindfulness of this feeling and its implications for real life that is a key precondition of the parent's ethically responding to the child as Other. Such a guilt-ridden parent, guilt-ridden in the positive sense of a mindfully-embraced genuine guilt, will, thus, ask himself searching questions: "What can I learn from my child? How might I better respond to the child's summoning 'command?' How can I be, better be, for the child?" (Todd, 2003, pp. 117–139). Such an orientation to one's child reflects the very responsible subjectivity of parenting at its best.

Conclusion

We have focused on some of the ethical preconditions, processes, and psychodynamics associated with good parenting, these being important in assisting one's child to flourish as a human being capable of love and work and moral probity. However, the main focus of this chapter has been to show in what way wanting, having, and raising a child, enlarges and deepens the ethicality of the parent. We have discussed a number of important elements that create the conditions of possibility for the parent to become a better parent and person, someone whose way of being in the world is mainly for-the-Other before himself, Levinas's definition of goodness.

That being said, it is important to note that, in the real world, most parents are not motivated towards goodness for entirely selfless reasons. As Freud has pointed out, there is always some kind of narcissistic "payoff" for any so-called selfless act. This self-enhancement could be the good feeling of living according to one's values. For the parent, however, I believe that there is one special narcissistic gain that is an important contributor to what makes many parents want to give to their children until it hurts, and that is the fear of abandonment, of losing their child's love and respect. Indeed, this is an often overlooked psychological aspect of the ethical relation between a parent and his child, one that reflects a primordial wish for connection and togetherness, a manifestation of ethicality that is implicit in this relation in the first place. Parents, in other words, fear their children's judgement of them in at least two ways: first, in the sense that their children correctly blame them for some of their own failures and limitations (and, in other instances, unjustly). This kind of accusation from a child in whatever form it takes is deeply painful to most thoughtful parents because there is almost always a trace of truth in it. However, in a certain sense, it is not as bad as the parent's self-awareness that his children—"so promising in youth, so much the mainstay of his life"—did not reach their own full potential (Weinstein, 1998, p. 23). This can be a reminder of the parent's own failures, of just how flawed he is, not only in the eyes of his children, but, more painfully, in his own eyes. (I am not including in this characterization those dreams on the part of the parent for the child that are based on the parent's wishes for the child to compensate for the parents' own inadequacies and failures in their lives.) As Arthur Miller showed so brilliantly in *Death of a Salesman*, "time and life are" pitiless "in their undoing of dreams" (*ibid*. p. 23), and children are often the "quintessential dream of life" (*ibid*., p. 28). It is the parent's awareness of his role in his child's undoing, of her not getting on in her life, that often haunts the parent; whether reasonable or not (the latter because, in a certain sense, our emotional lives have a strange autonomy, an "otherness" that feels beyond our command [*ibid*., p. 25]). In a sense, from a Levinasian point of view, and this is the pathos of parenting, "time and life", our children, "betray us, erode our promise" (*ibid*., p. 29), just as we inevitably fail them. There is, in other words, a peculiar form of the tragic that is inevitable in the parent–child relation. This, too, when fully embraced constitutes the ethical potential of the parent–child love relation. The question is: why?

The answer to this question is that with such an awareness of the tragic element in the parent–child relation, the parent will be motivated to do better, to be more caring, more serving, and more being for the child before himself. This includes within it the capacity to say "No", to set appropriate limits, even when this takes more effort than simply giving in to the child. Infinite compassion is an infinite obligation, says Levinas. In a certain sense, to use an admittedly extreme, though evocatively apt analogy, as with the religious person who apprehends his estrangement from God, who feels guilty that he has failed his God, there is often within his soul a mysterious irruption of conscience, a deep wish, felt as a command, to better "love, fear, and serve" God. It is precisely this triad of elements, in part rooted in an upsurge of genuine guilt, that often propels the good parent to want to do better for his child, to relate to him with a similar worshipful inner attitude, with devotion and respect, as with the man trying to find his way back to God. Indeed, love of God—that passionate "longing and yearning" for "nearness" to Him, the "bliss and delight" in occupying oneself with Him; fear of God—that "grateful reverence", that "loving fear", as Herman Cohen called it, which leads a man to "cling" to God, to want to serve Him; and service to God—the mindful dedication of all one's actions in the mundane world to serve God, especially through kindness—these are the touchstones, the royal road to God, Goodness, and to good parenting (Hertz, 1960, pp. 770, 790, 984). Indeed, as the ancient Rabbis have repeatedly noted, for the person—in our context, the parent—who embraces such way of being, his life, and more importantly, his child's life, will be worthy of a Divine blessing.

CHAPTER SEVEN

On feeling altogether miserable: getting help through psychotherapy

> "But my life now, my whole life, independently of anything that can happen to me, every minute of it is no longer meaningless as it was before, but has a positive meaning of goodness with which I have the power to invest it"
>
> Leo Tolstoy

There is a certain truth to Frank Sinatra's pithy remark—"I'm for anything that can get you through the night, be it prayer, tranquillizers or a bottle of Jack Daniels." Sinatra was correctly putting his finger on something that most of us know by the time we are adults: that life can be frustrating and harsh, if not painful, much of the time; at least that is the sense that some of us have when we let ourselves honestly reflect on the matter. "Man's existential condition," says one philosopher, "means suffering, doubt, struggles with the world and within oneself" (Peli, 1984, p. 18). As is common knowledge, learning how to quietly endure a degree of pain is a sign of maturity, and sometimes it is a great catalyst for life, that is, for living life better. Sinatra was also insinuating a deeper point; he was noting that when one is feeling miserable, one wants to feel better fast, which often leads us to do just about anything to make the distress go away. However, for some people, prayer, a tranquillizer, or a bottle of Jack Daniels or its equivalent, will not do the trick, at least not in a sustained way, and these wise and courageous (and sometimes desperate) people decide that it is time to get some professional help. Often, the helper is a psychotherapist, someone who is trained to assist the person to feel better and get on with his or her life in a more productive way.

There are, of course, a mind-boggling array of different types of psychotherapy—usually defined, at least most basically, as "the treatment of mental disorders by psychological methods"—available to the average person who is in distress. In general, depending on what one's problem in living is, it is appropriate to find a specialist, or at least someone very experienced in treating that kind of problem. For example, if one suffers from a discrete symptom, such as premature ejaculation with one's loved wife or significant other, it would probably be more sensible to go to a cognitive-behaviour sex therapist than to a Freudian psychoanalyst (even though the problem has to do with sex!). Premature ejaculation, if it does signify a more deep-seated intimacy problem in the man (or couple), can be corrected in ten or so sessions in contrast to the man's spending a number of years with an analyst like myself, with little guarantee that the presenting problem will be corrected. Likewise, with a marital problem related to how one raises one's children, or a public speaking phobia, it is better to go to a therapist who deals with such issues on an everyday basis than to go to someone who simply dabbles in marital counselling or phobia work.

Unfortunately, most of the problems of living that people go to a psychotherapist for are not nearly so simple to treat as premature ejaculation, conflicts over parenting styles, or the fear of speaking in large groups. There is a wide range of patients who suffer from certain types of amorphous anxiety and/or depressive conditions whose origins are hard to pin down (i.e., nothing in the external world has obviously caused the condition, including its magnitude), and the correction of which is hardly straightforward. The reason for this is that the anxiety and depression, while symptomatically troubling, and, to a certain extent, suppressible by psychotropic medications like Paxil or Lexapro, are not the *real* problems. Rather, such people's suffering emanates from complex unconscious sources, usually rooted in their childhood, as well as internalized conflicts and early personal deficits, which still have a strong emotional grip on how they relate to themselves and to others. These mostly unconscious conflicts, deficits, and the like determine their outlook and the way they live their everyday lives, despite their best intentions to have it otherwise. Such patients recognize that their thoughts, feelings, and actions are unreasonable, that they simply do not make any sense. Such patients may or may not want to use medication to feel better (and I am not against medication, it is great when it works), but they are often strongly motivated to get to the root of their problem. As Freud wrote, "The primary motive force in the therapy is the patient's suffering and the wish to be cured that arises from it" (Freud, 1913c, p. 143). Thus, at least ideally, armed with new self-understandings and insights, these patients make the necessary changes in their perspective and behaviour to have a decent shot at having the better life they want.

This chapter strives to show what a Levinasian-inspired, ethically-infused psychoanalytic psychotherapy can uniquely offer the patient who suffers from anxiety and depression (technically, an agitated depression, a mixture of anxiety and depression), and other types of problems in living that are not usually part of the normative account of psychoanalytic treatment (a treatment modality that was once common in popular culture, though now is often mistakenly criticized as outdated). Whether one goes to a psychoanalyst or another kind of so-called insight-orientated psychotherapist or "talking cure", the fact is that Levinas's main focus, the ethical domain—being responsive and responsible to and for the Other, often before oneself—is perhaps the crucial, often overlooked, condition of possibility for desirable deep self-transformation and, for that matter, symptom-reduction. In a word, I am talking about enhancing a patient's sense of overall happiness, happiness being defined *not* simply as it is usually construed, as feeling or showing transient pleasure, contentment, or joy. Rather, or should I say, in addition to these praiseworthy states of being, I am referring to Freud's words about the possibility of achieving a modicum of happiness in this crazy world: the goal of analysis, he famously said, was "to convert neurotic misery into ordinary unhappiness". In other words, given the harshness of the human condition as most of us experience it in Western society, the individual and society are, in a certain sense, at odds with each other; as Freud showed, we are destined, at least from time to time, to feel anguish—"I suffer, therefore I am". While some may think such an observation is a pessimistic overstatement, the great church father St Augustine, who more or less agreed with Freud on this point, put his finger on an aspect of life as many of us experience it: from the cradle to the grave it is a distress-filled existence. Happiness, in other words, is not a fixed end point, let alone a permanent, or even semi-permanent state of mind, but, rather, it is the episodically-sensed by-product of living the so-called "good life". Freud, St Augustine and Levinas would probably all agree on this point.

This chapter will be structured around three practical questions that are pertinent to the patient/analyst encounter; coincidentally, these are the same questions that I, and most car owners, ask their mechanic when they take their car in for a repair: "What's the problem?", "How did it get there?", and "How can we fix it?" (and, of course, perhaps most importantly, how much will it cost?—in personal effort, self-confrontation, and struggle). Finally, a case vignette of an extraordinary man I treated (and still treat), initially presenting with an agitated depression (and many other serious problems), will be described to illustrate some of the theoretical points made in the first part of the chapter and to give a real-life feel to how a Levinasian-inspired, ethically-infused psychoanalytic psychotherapy works.

What is the problem (or, how does the analyst conceptualize the patient's presenting problem)?

In psychoanalytic thought, personality or character is defined in a well-known textbook as "the enduring, patterned functioning of an individual ... it is the person's habitual way of thinking, feeling and acting ... the person's habitual mode of reconciling intrapsychic conflicts" (Moore & Fine, 1990, p. 37). This standard definition is useful to the clinician, but it leaves out what I think is most important, which is the ethical nature of the person. In this Levinasian view, personality becomes "a point where responsibility is concentrated". That is, personality is best understood as "moral personality", as a subjectivity that comprehends itself as responsibility for the other (Wyschogrod, 2000, p. 125). This place where responsibility is concentrated is a kind of "resource for moral recognition", "ethically sound practical reasoning", and, ultimately, moral "recovery" or repossession of ourselves (Jacobs, 2001, p. 43). In other words, personality or character can be viewed as the action-guiding nexus for enacting our moral values, for responsibility for the other. In this view, a personality or character disorder, at least most generally, can be defined as the habitual conscious and unconscious ways that a person is inadequately responsive, misguided, and or deaf to ethical considerations, to the summoning call of the Other as one's normative horizon of feeling, thought, and action.

For example, in the narcissistic personality disorder, the person's habitual way of perceiving, relating to, and thinking about the other is marked by grandiosity, envy, and an inordinate need for admiration. Such an outlook cuts him off from properly empathizing with, and responding to, the reasonable needs and desires of the other. Instead, the other is exploited to advance his own ends, to have his excessive need for self-aggrandizement, self-importance, and specialness affirmed again and again. The borderline personality, who has marked lability in his sense of self, emotions, and impulse control, has volatile, unstable, and explosive interpersonal relationships that make it nearly impossible to consider the other's needs and wishes in any sustained and reasonable manner. His fear of abandonment, his inordinate need for idealization and quick sense of devaluation, his boundless rage, all diminish, if not arrest, his ability to give and receive love. Likewise, the mode of being in the world of the antisocial personality can also be fruitfully analysed in terms of its ethical meaning and significance, as evidenced in the individual's diminished capacity to respond empathetically to the other's needs for love and justice. The antisocial's harmful, disruptive, inconsiderate interpersonal approach, always at the expense of the other's rights and needs, is his distinguishing feature. In all of these and other personality disorders, the individual is ethically corrupted, unable to respond with the fullness of his whole being to the reasonable needs and desires of the other in an ethically healthy, genuinely other-regarding manner. As a result of their truncated ties to empathy, those analysands with personality or character disorders, whether they acknowledge it or not, are suffering greatly, for they reside in a loveless hell.

Needless to say, by the time a person, including those patients with the personality disorders described above, decides to seek professional help, he is usually in a pretty bad state of mind and his life is often way off track. Whether such individuals are jumping out of their skins with anxiety, or are weighed down by depression, whether their marriage is imploding, whether they are at war with their "acting out" teenager, or are about to be fired from their job, such people are mainly driven by a wish to reduce their anguish, to find a way out of their loveless hell, whether that be with one's spouse, significant other, children, boss, or whomever.

From a Levinasian point of view, what is striking about all patients who come for help is that they feel inescapably riveted to their anguish. It feels and looks to them as if there is "no exit" from their distressing emotional experience and real-life situation. It is this "failure to find an escape from self-absorption" that is typical of intense anxiety, depression, and all other debilitating, painful conditions of the mind and heart (Cohen, 2005, p. 111). Levinas makes this point when he says, "escape is the need to get out of oneself, that is, to break that most radical and unalterably binding of chains, the fact that the I is oneself" (Levinas, 2003, p. 55). In other words, regardless of the specific reasons why a patient seeks out an analyst, regardless of his unique familial history and psychodynamics, the common substructure to his presenting problem, at least from a Levinasian point of view, is that he feels utterly trapped in his own psychological skin; he wants to find an exit from his current "self", "I", "Ego" experience. In a word, he wants to be otherwise than who he is. "Otherwise than being", Levinas calls this move out of a narcissistic prison towards the other, in responsibility.

So, for example, the patient who feels pervasive anxiety—that awful nervousness or agitation, often about something bad that is going to happen, or that state of intense apprehension or fear of real or imagined danger—is usually utterly self-consuming. Such a person may occasionally have a moment of respite; however, the rest of the time he feels almost entirely consumed by surges of preoccupying anxious feelings that seem never to end. The horror of this way of being was strikingly brought home to me when a patient of mine, an ex-Marine, told me that when he recently flew to England on vacation with his wife, from the moment he got off the plane in London until he returned home ten days later, he was in a full-blown panic. Phobic about taking any psychiatric medication, and not wanting to upset his wife by ruining their vacation, he somehow endured what he described as the worst ten days of his life, suffering alone in silence. What this patient did tell me that is especially relevant to our current discussion was that, despite his putting on a front to the outside world, including to his wife, "There was not one second when I was not horrifyingly aware of the panic I was feeling . . . I was more afraid than when I was being shot at in downtown Baghdad." While admittedly an extreme example, this man was testifying to what Levinas was getting at when he described the "there is", that radically unsettling feeling of anonymous and impersonal being, characterized by being riveted to oneself, imprisoned in a state of terrifying, inescapable self-absorption.

Similarly, as any depressed patient will tell you, he feels trapped in his way of being in the world. Depression—those relentless feelings of hopelessness, dejection, poor concentration, lack of energy, inability to sleep, and, sometimes, suicidal tendencies—is known to be highly narcissistic. The depressed person feels almost totally self-centred, full of himself, at times reaching out to others, though often for pity, a pity that psychoanalyst Theodore Reik said one should never give during treatment, "No *rachmones* [pity] for depressives!" That is because pity only feeds the depressive's false consciousness, his infantile wish to be rescued without having to do the heavy work of facing himself, especially his anger and hostility, and his wish to manipulate others into taking care of him. Moreover, says Reik, pity is often given for the wrong reasons, to make oneself, the analyst, feel better. Thus, whether it is anxiety, depression, or a mixture of the two, the important point is that both conditions are utterly self-absorbing, if not self-cannibalizing, and this feature is what the Levinasian-inspired analyst (all analysts in my view) needs to be mindful of if he is to help the patient free himself from himself. According to Nietzsche, such self-overcoming is a form of spiritual development, one that distinguishes the "slave" from the "master", the "bound spirit" from the "free spirit." It is the difference between feeling hopeless or hopeful.

How did the problem develop (or, how did I get to feel so horrible and mess up my life so badly)?

It is common knowledge among psychoanalysts that every patient comes to his condition by way of a highly idiosyncratic trajectory rooted in his personal history and psychodynamics. Although there are quasi-determinative motivational patterns that an analyst tends to see over and over again, the fact is that these general causal patterns and their corresponding theoretical notions are only relatively helpful in understanding and helping a patient find his way out of himself, to move from loveless hell to authentic love, conceived as responsibility for the Other, often before oneself.

For Levinas, analysands' problems in living and psychopathology are best understood in terms of their being "ethically disabled". As Jacobs observes, their mode of being in the world, "their characters, are such that sound ethical considerations" (Jacobs, 2001, p. 1), the for the Other of responsibility, are largely "inaccessible to them". Moreover, such analysands have a seriously restricted capacity for moral self-transformation, "for ethical self-correction" (*ibid.*, p. 74). In Levinasian language, an ethically disabled analysand is more or less consistently and significantly estranged from the Good. Such an analysand can be said to lack ethical integrity and "good" character, the "irreproachable character" that Freud believed was a prerequisite to being a competent treating analyst (Freud, 1905[1904], p. 267). Not surprisingly, the main reasons for this ethical disablement are almost always rooted in one's childhood experience of being parented, parents being the "usual suspects" who contribute to a person's becoming truncated in his ability to love and work. While there are infinite permutations of such imperfect parenting, from classic neglect and abuse to less extreme forms of inadequate parenting, the fact is that what is common to all of these experiences, at least on the most elemental level, is that the child felt insufficiently and inadequately loved, sometimes traumatically so. Such self-deficits, commonly experienced as extreme emptiness and unsettledness, are among the necessary psychological prerequisites for the child to become an adult who is self-obsessed, and who views others mainly in instrumental terms. "What's in it for me?" and "What is best for me?" are the watchwords of such people. In a nutshell, such people tend to be mainly self-directed and self-regarding (in the negative sense), rather than other-directed and other-regarding (the Levinasian ideal).

Put differently, in general, to the extent that the natural inclination of the self, the ego, towards selfishness dominates one's life, especially in one's interpersonal relations, one is more likely to suffer guilt, anxiety, depression, and alienation. It is important to recognize, however, that the Levinasian subject, in a fundamental sense, acts according to spontaneous selfishness, that the subject is basically egotistical. In fact, egotism is not a despicable flaw on the part of the subject, but the subject's very nature (Smith, 2005, pp. 147, 150, 256). "Egotism is not an ugly vice on the part of the subject, but its ontology . . ." (Levinas, 1996b, pp. 70–71). This view is very much in harmony with Nietzsche, who wrote, "Selfishness is not a principle, but the sole and unique fact" (Assoun, 2000, p. 75), and with Freud, who observed, "Narcissism is the universal and original state of things, from which object-love is only later developed, without the narcissism necessarily disappearing on that account" (Freud, 1916–1917, p. 416). Levinas, the Holocaust survivor, is no innocent; he understands that the self can never be completely modified in that it is inherently "for itself", that is, selfish and self-referential. Levinas evocatively makes this point when he writes, "No one is good voluntarily. No one is enslaved to the Good" (Levinas, 1998b, p. 11). And elsewhere he notes that "responsibility for the other is the good. It is not pleasant, it is good" (Robbins, 2001, p. 47). Levinas, like Freud and his followers, recognizes that overcoming, even significantly modulating, our inherent selfishness, infantile narcissism, and tendency towards egocentricity is very difficult.

What Levinas is suggesting is that a human being in his ethical expression is an exception to selfishness, infantile narcissism, and egocentricity, to this central striving in existence, "to preserve oneself in being" (*conatus essendi*), as Spinoza called it (Smith, 2005, p. 65.) There is an alternative mode of being worth moving towards, the search for "the Good" that is beyond being (i.e., following Plato, everything, including Being, is to be apprehended in terms of the Good). This "otherwise than being" is depicted, for example, in the biblical/prophetic tradition in Judaism, in which ethics is its very centre, and in all of the ancient religious wisdom traditions. Saints, *tzadikkim* (righteous people), and all those who live lives of holiness, of radical selflessness and kindness, characterize the otherwise than being that Levinas has in mind.

Thus, many problems in living, and, in their extreme, psychopathology, emanate in part from the selfish self undermining, if not taking over, the ethical self. The needs and aspirations of the selfish self, the ego, have priority over the life-affirming needs of the other. When the ego is tied to the self in this manner, the fundamental isolation and loneliness of the subject remains continuous and steady. Psychoanalysis, with its interest in narcissistic pathologies, has provided much insight into the development and tragic course of such a way of being. For Levinas, to the extent that one avoids and ignores one's responsibility for the other, including what we do carelessly, inadvertently, and unconsciously, one can be said to be ethically disabled, lacking what Levinas calls "humaneness". In one of his Talmudic discussions, he asks,

> To shelter the other in one's own land or home, to tolerate the presence of the landless and homeless on the ancestral soil, so jealously, so meanly loved—is that the criterion of humanness? Unquestionably so. [Levinas, 1994, p, 98]

The above extract speaks to Levinas's criterion for the ethical life, infinite responsibility, and compassion in the form of responding with the fullness of one's being to the life-affirming material, psychological, or spiritual needs of the other. Says Levinas, "Sociality, for me [the for-the-Other that commands the I], is the best of the human" (Levinas, 2000b, p. 103). Pathology, so to speak, can be conceptualized as those habits of mind, heart, and behaviour that impede the movement of transcendence, away from being, towards living a life characterized by love and justice for the other before oneself. Indeed, from a Levinasian point of view, a person's capacity for critical, ethical self-reflection, acknowledging when moral requirements and obligations to the Other have not been properly met and responded to, is a good prognostic indicator for a successful analysis.

In mainstream psychoanalytic terms, the above refers to the transmutation of narcissism from infantile to more mature forms and the development of deep and wide-ranging emotional capacities for empathy, compassion, and love. Psychoanalysis has been masterful in its ability to describe, understand, and ameliorate the many developmental and conflictual impediments that blunt, impair, and block individuals' capacity to live a life guided by love and justice, as Levinas defines those terms. Thus, love is conceived as responsibility to, and for, the Other and justice, working for the kind-hearted "peaceful resolution of infinite responsibilities" for the other, and secondarily, the satisfaction of my interests and rights (Hutchens, 2004, p. 99).

How to fix the problem (or, how do I transform myself so that I can serve the Other in love and justice)?

Once one knows what one's problem is (inordinate narcissism), and how it developed from parental inadequacies (and other traumas) that created an unsustainable needy, selfish self, the most difficult aspect of any analytic treatment is how to "fix" the problem, how to bring about deep self-transformation, the kind of self-change that often leads to a sense of self-transcendence, that also tends to correlate with a feeling of greater overall happiness.

For a Levinasian-inspired analyst, the way to achieve such self-transformation involves the patient making a commitment to shaping a new conception of the self, one that moves against the self-encapsulated, intensely self-serving individualism that is so common in our Western society. Put differently, the patient needs to awaken "to a moral life" that is coterminous "with the discovery that the other is the first to be" valued, appreciated, "served" (Peperzak, 1993, p. 111). It is the development of a moral consciousness, defined as the mindfulness of "the privilege the other has relative to me", that characterizes a successful analysis. (*ibid.*, p. 112). Only when there has been a self-transfiguration "of a being-for-itself into a being-for-the-other through moral responsibility and obligation" (Cohen, 2002, p. 60), in a sense, an unchosen, undeclinable obligation emanating from "my condition as a subject", in which "I am given over to the Other" (Davis, 1996, p. 81), has the analysand reached the end of analysis. Paraphrasing Freud, a Levinasian-inspired psychoanalysis, with its demand for infinite responsibility and obligation to the Other—there is always more giving and serving to do—makes analysis, in a certain sense, interminable.

The resulting reduction of inordinate and infantile narcissism, on the way to "otherwise than being", Levinas was well aware of. In fact, as Smith points out (Smith, 2005, pp. 12, 42, 104), Levinas viewed the undoing or emptying out of the selfish self, the naturally egotistical I, as it is ethically solicited, summoned by the other in responsibility, as the prerequisite for "otherwise than being". The imprisonment of self within itself, and its tendency to assimilate otherness to itself, by knowledge, possession, and mastery, needs to be gradually challenged, disrupted, and ultimately emptied out and then transformed by the other, by being hostage to the other. It is, says Smith, through an "unselving or transselving", by being roused, stirred, and troubled by the other that one moves towards the Good, Goodness, "to-God" that is to the transcendent state of being "for the Other". Such an approach is entirely in keeping with those all too few psychoanalytic theorists who wisely argue that it is the development of a "non-self-centric subjectivity" that should be the main goal of any psychoanalysis (Rubin, 1996, pp. 8, 190; Marcus, 2003, pp. 52, 185–188). To some extent, mainstream psychoanalysis recognizes this point when it distinguishes so-called "normal narcissism" as manifested in ample self-care, level-headed self-confidence, and reasonable self-regard from "heightened narcissism", as expressed in conceit and smugness, a demand to be treated specially, a haughty sense of superiority over others, or utter grandiosity (Person, Cooper, & Gabbard, 2005, p. 555). To help an analysand achieve a modicum of happiness, probably the best we can do is to help him transform his selfish cravings and infantile narcissism into "Goodness".

In this context, the role of the analyst is to expand the analysand's awareness and understanding of what conscious and unconscious personal factors (e.g., thoughts, feelings, wishes, and fantasies) and, especially, valuative commitments impede, diminish, or take the place of an ethic of responsibility for the Other, as well as for oneself. (I have drawn liberally on Jacobs, *Choosing Character* [2001], for the following comments.) This includes, for example: (1) deconstructing the many ways that analysands deceive themselves, defend and insulate themselves against feeling appropriate guilt, shame, remorse, and self-reproach for their misdeeds towards others; (2) understanding why the analysand is unmoved to reflect on and re-evaluate his selfish and immoral acts, or even perceive that he has acted selfishly or hurtfully towards others. This involves analysing the analysand's valuative attachments, especially within the context of their personal background and moral history, including the vulnerability, anxiety, pain, confusion, and conflict that almost always sustain misguided valuative attachments and self-serving behaviour; (3) understanding why the analysand is often unmoved by constructive criticisms of his immoral actions and associated feelings and thoughts, why they do not self-correct. The analyst needs to help the analysand work through his conscious reasons and unconscious motivations for willingly causing suffering to others, for being unjust in his relationships. This means encouraging the analysand to see how his various moral lapses, often rooted in interference by his selfishness and inordinate desire for self-affirmation and gratification, make his own and his loved one's lives miserable.

Thus, we can say that, in such a Levinasian-inspired form of psychoanalysis, we are always doing "character analysis", the aim of which is to help the analysand recognize and deeply appreciate ethical considerations, being-for-the-Other. Most importantly, this means being motivated by such a valuative action-guiding commitment, towards living what in theological circles is called a virtuous life. In a Levinasian-glossed psychoanalytic language, this means helping the analysand become a morally autonomous and integrated individual, one who has the effective cognitive, emotional, and motivational capacity to be stably devoted and attached to the Good, a life devoted less to questing after fame and fortune and more to service to others. Responsibility for others thus becomes the fundamental meaning of self-identity.

Before we move to the illustrative case vignette, let us summarize by returning to the three main questions concerning psychopathology that began this chapter: What is the problem?—radical self-absorption, a self that is mainly, if not utterly, "for-itself"; How did the problem develop?—parental inadequacies in childhood, and other harmful-to the-self experiences that helped create a selfish self with inordinate narcissistic needs; How to fix the problem?—moving the analysand from a being that is "for-itself" to one that is "responsible for-the-Other".

Case vignette

Vincent is a fifty-nine-year-old, physically huge, extremely affable Italian man raised in a rough section of Brooklyn, the son of abusive and neglectful parents: his authoritarian father owned a butcher shop/delicatessen, while his "refrigerator" mother hated working there as the behind-the-scenes cook. Vincent is a retired insurance salesman/supervisor who first came to me about fifteen years ago in an extremely bad emotional state, actually on the edge of a nervous breakdown.

Vincent, who had been married six times, had had an incident involving his most recently divorced wife, a sexy German blonde who worked in the same office as he did. Originally her supervisor, he seduced her (including "screwing" her on his office desk), married her, and legally separated from her a few months later, while the official divorce was in process. Apparently, his ex-wife was being "hit on" by Vincent's regional boss. Vincent became so enraged when he saw his boss kiss his ex-wife on the neck that, in a fit of jealous fury, he verbally cursed him and then picked him up over his head like a bar-bell and threatened to throw him through the window of the high-rise building where they worked. Security was called, Vincent was removed from the building and subsequently fired. However, the insurance company, in order to avoid public scandal, a scandal that Vincent threatened to make, as he was aware of a number of unofficially sanctioned illegal dealings going on in his office involving a great deal of stolen money, agreed to a very generous severance arrangement based, in part, on documentation from me that Vincent was mentally unfit to return to work. Indeed, I believed Vincent when he told me that if he had to return to work, he could not take any criticism, let alone orders from anyone, and if forced to return to earning a living, he would most assuredly violently erupt at some point: "If they make me go back, or if I have to work again, I will kill someone, I know it." The insurance company wisely decided that it was not worth the risk and paid Vincent to disappear. Vincent has been living well on his severance pay, his savings, his successful investments, and, for the last decade or so, from his seventh wife's excellent salary. Incidentally, Vincent has one child from his first wife, now a young adult, and he impressed me as a fairly good father overall, though they had very hard times during his son's adolescence (which were mostly Vincent's fault, rooted in his unreasonable narcissistic need to force his son to his will). Moreover, his first wife, the mother of his son, viewed Vincent as a "great guy", a dutiful ex-husband and a responsible father. I had met her once some considerable time previously when their son was having some problems. In fact, his first wife bakes him Christmas cookies, which behaviour, in the pained world of divorce, is unusual.

When Vincent first came to me he was "lean and mean", as he described himself. In fact he looked strikingly similar to a young Steven Segal, pony tail, cool attire, the whole get up. At the time he came to me, he had been whoring around for nearly twenty years, having slept with an incredible number of women (he estimated about three thousand, including some famous actresses!), he drank a quart of Scotch a day, smoked like a chimney, and fiercely exercised to keep his attractive "macho" appearance intact. Though he took his insurance work seriously (he was one of most successful insurance salesman in the company's history), and was a dedicated father (when he had visitation with his son he was with him 24/7), Vincent spent most of his off-time hitting the high-end Manhattan bars, where he was regarded as something of a celebrity. Genial, generous, a superb storyteller, and altogether great fun to be around, especially when intoxicated—"drinking brought the best out of me, it released my goodness. I became everyone's Teddy Bear"—Vincent derived enormous gratification from his nightlife of wine, women and song. That he typically only needed three hours of sleep a night to adequately function in his ordinary life made his spirited nightlife possible.

For some reason, all of this came crashing down. Somewhat like Tony Soprano, Vincent began to develop episodic anxiety attacks and strange depressive feelings, feelings he said he had never felt before. "Even a quart of Scotch a day and fucking my brains out could not make those shitty feelings go away," he said. After trying to exercise his condition away (Vincent had greatly increased his already rigorous exercise regime, even once jogging by the seashore during a hurricane, while "shadow boxing with the waves"), he finally capitulated to his best friend's advice to seek professional help. He got my name from an ex-policeman I had treated. I was the third therapist Vincent had seen, the other two having been found from his insurance plan; they "bored and annoyed me, the last guy made me feel like I was fuckin' crazy . . . I was being cheap, I knew it would never work out, because none of the others were 'Jewish doctors'." As will become clear shortly, Vincent had a special connection to Jewish doctors, rooted in his own traumatic childhood illness, in which a German Jewish doctor saved his life.

When I first met Vincent, I found him to have a commanding presence. He was very articulate and interesting to listen to, actually a charming master of conversation who loved holding forth. This was not altogether surprising, as he was a college graduate who had completed one year of law school before dropping out. During the first few sessions, Vincent told me about his mostly legal gun collection, which was worth about $50,000, his Rolls Royce, his being a gourmet chef, his love of hunting and fishing, his building with his own hands an authentic English pub in his basement, and, perhaps his most secret yearning, his love of the English aristocracy, which he fantasized becoming a member of. I had received my PhD at the University of London (my diploma was on my wall), and my wife was English, though Jewish English, not exactly the "right" pedigree, but still. She also often answered my work phone. All those things further endeared me to Vincent as we worked together.

Though Vincent was easy to converse with, he was by no means an easy patient to engage on an emotionally meaningful level, especially initially. He was, for example, controlling. If I was as little as one minute late for his session, he would slip the cheque under the door and go home, feeling I had disrespected him. In his mind, since he was always on time (only once in fifteen years had he been late, the result of a traffic jam), he always paid at the session, and he easily accommodated his schedule to any schedule changes I asked for, he deserved to be seen on time as he wanted. Needless to say, psychologically speaking, there was more to all this, but Vincent hardly gave way over the years despite my numerous psychoanalytic interpretations. Now, fortunately, he can be kept waiting for three minutes (he is hovering by the door), so long as I tell him that I will be a minute or two late and apologize for keeping him waiting. I have been well trained!

Vincent could also be downright intimidating. His effort at intimidation emerged early on when he came to the session with two large violin-shaped cases. He said that he wanted to show me a few things, opened the first case and took out a beautiful, hand-carved elephant gun. Pointing out its details, Vincent sensed my great interest and appreciation for this work of art, as I called it. Returning to my chair, I then heard Vincent indicating that he wanted to show me something from the other case. He took out another gun; however, this time it was a German assault rifle. Standing next to the window, Vincent put the gun in my hands, and asked me what I thought about this "monster gun". I hesitated, and he then took the gun back and proceeded to put in a live clip and cock it, an ominous sound that is still hard to forget. For a moment I had a tinge of anxiety, interestingly, not about my being killed (I guess I was in denial), but that he was going to shoot into the many pedestrians underneath my window overlooking a busy Queens Boulevard intersection. Said Vincent, stroking the gun, "It's terrifying isn't it?" I said, "Yes." Vincent then leaned closer to me and said, "Now, tell me, Doc, when the niggers come through the windows, do you want to greet them with a baseball bat or this baby?" I looked into Vincent's intense eyes and said, "Well, when you put it that way, I would rather have the assault rifle." Said a smiling Vincent, "That's why I really like you Doc, you're the first shrink who has ever made me feel that my love of guns is normal!" I cracked a nervous smile, and said, "I am glad you feel that way Vincent" (to myself, I said, this situation is insane, as my empathy had had the troubling unintended consequence of normalizing this guy). Although I wanted to "join" with Vincent, to express real interest in his world of meaning, that of gun culture, I did not want to make him feel that his obsession with guns, with the violence they signified, was a good thing. In any event, this interchange was a pivotal one for our relationship, for Vincent had essentially told me that he felt understood and supported, not judged, and, most importantly, for this Italian man, he felt respected, and respectful, as I was not a wimp. Subsequent to this interchange, Vincent occasionally gave me magazines about guns that I read with increasing interest, as it was an intriguing "man's" world I was unfamiliar with. He also encouraged me to buy a shotgun for home protection (in fact, later on I did get a licensed hand-gun for protection, as I was seriously threatened by a patient, information Vincent found out when he once noticed my concealed gun during a session). Needless to say, Vincent was pleased I had taken his advice.

Returning to the first of our three organizing questions of this chapter, "What's the problem?", that is, what was the initial meaning of Vincent's anxious and depressive symptoms?, it is always best to consider first how the patient views his own problems in living. Briefly, though in general Vincent was very articulate and street savvy about sizing up people, he was utterly bewildered by the workings of his own anxious and depressed mind. In fact, he told me that he had never been so clueless about his inner workings as he was now. As I told him, in a way this was good, because, unless he felt ambushed, or at least troubled by his own unintelligible feelings and thoughts, that is "disrupted", he would never have taken the time to take a look at how he had been living. Agreeing, he told me that he thought his anxious and depressing feelings were associated with the blow to his ego that his ex-wife's affair had caused him: "The cunt betrayed me, she made me look like the ultimate loser, kissing that 'nigger cock sucker' by the water fountain, the whole office saw it." Recasting Vincent's formulation in straightforward psychological terms, he felt severely narcissistically wounded by what he viewed as his wife's disrespect and disloyalty to him, an assault on his manhood that he could not tolerate. Feeling nearly castrated, his masculine self-image being severely compromised, and publicly at that, and being furious about it with no adequate outlet, caused him severe anxiety. His anxiety attacks represented his failed attempts to control his rage at his disrespecting wife, a woman who, in one fell swoop, had subverted his tenuous macho-based world of meaning. Moreover, Vincent's depressive feelings, his periodically feeling like a deflated balloon, were associated with his turning his rage on himself. As will become clear later, while these clinical formulations were basically true, they were only the tip of the iceberg in terms of understanding what Vincent was *really* dealing with, that is, his childhood traumas.

Thus, we can answer our question, "What was Vincent's problem?" by saying he was a man who was extremely narcissistically vulnerable, especially to insult or criticism. His self-esteem and self-concept were insecurely based; he was even self-hating, and thus he was vulnerable to emotional storms, to feeling like an empty vessel or a raging bull. Excessive alcohol, smoking, food, whoring around, hitting the clubs and the like, were his desperate ways of filling himself up, while at the same time these activities muted his rage. Where did these painful affects come from?

I mentioned that Vincent came from an abusive home, emanating from both his parents. This was confirmed when I met his older brother, who was having marital problems, and whose stories of mistreatment by his parents were similar to Vincent's, though not nearly as bad.

Indeed, Vincent had a classically abusive father—explosive, unreasonably critical, mean-spirited, and emotionally remote. "What do you want to hear Doc? About the time I was thrown across the living room into a door so hard that its hinges were ripped off. Or when I was thrown down the stairs, or when my balls were slammed into the vanity, or getting the shit beaten out of me for no good reason. Plain and simple, it was a fuckin' horror show in my house." Thus, said Vincent, early on he learned how to stay out of the line of fire, at least most of the time. Above all, he never disrespected his father, and that meant being completely compliant. That Vincent had felt utterly controlled and submissive, and now in his adult life cannot tolerate any controls that he deems unreasonable, for example, if I am a few minutes late for a session, or he has to complete a stupid form for some bureaucracy, is not entirely surprising. Waiting and/or being requested, in his mind, "ordered", to do something stupid brings back the impotent rage that Vincent says he felt during most of his childhood. Impotent rage, or any similar feeling that smacks of subjugation, is a key issue for Vincent, a feeling he cannot tolerate as an adult. However, when he can express this rage for a righteous cause, he almost always takes action. Once, for example, he saw an elderly Black woman being mugged and robbed on the street by a young, knife-wielding, drugged-out thug. Vincent jumped out of his car, disarmed the thug who was pulling at the woman's handbag—actually he beat him unconscious—and returned the handbag. Said the elderly woman, "How can I thank you?" "Just forget I was ever here," answered Vincent, who nonchalantly walked to his car and drove away. Vincent said that on the night after the incident, "I slept like a baby." There were other instances when Vincent put himself in harm's way to help someone who was being mistreated, or when he felt he was being menaced. Said Vincent, "I *never* back off from a confrontation with a prick bully, *ever*." Unlike his behaviour when his father mistreated him, when, as an adult, Vincent's masculine self-respect was challenged, if not pummelled, he stood his ground; his integrity was non-negotiable. Such stories were instructive for me as well, for while I analysed the childhood basis for Vincent's fear of unreasonable control and criticism, including the impotent rage it evoked, I was able to be especially sensitive in my manner of dealing with him. There have only been two or three times in this long treatment when I was the target of his primitive rage, always verbally expressed. Because Vincent always wished to preserve me as essentially a "good" other, the treatment was never in danger of ending in a "hail of bullets". As Vincent once said to me, correctly, I often think, without the treatment he could, and would, get seriously off track in his life. "Vinny," I once playfully said, "we will grow old together." He nodded his head in agreement.

Vincent's mother was also a piece of work. From what he told me, she was cold, self-absorbed, critical, and, at times, downright nasty. One of Vincent's "favourite" memories for depicting just how bad his mother was was once when he came home from middle school, and during his walk home a flying bird had crapped on him, leaving a small dripping stain "the size of a dime" on his new jacket. When his mother saw him, she noticed the dripping stain and asked him what had happened. Vincent told the truth, that a flying bird had shit on him. His mother's reply was, "Why didn't you watch where you were walking!" She dragged him by his arm into the house and "beat the crap out of me".

Vincent said that there were many such instances, where his mother unreasonably held him responsible for ordinary mishaps, like spilling something or not wiping his feet well enough, in which no matter what he said, he was doomed to be severely yelled at or hit. "That bitch had a nasty mouth on her that could make hell freeze over," said Vinny. To make matters worse, Vinny spent *all* of his free time in childhood (including summers), from age eleven through his first year of law school—as "ordered" by his father, there was no choice—"rolling meatballs" in his father's delicatessen, sitting a few feet away from his profusely sweating, endlessly complaining mother, who was cooking over a hot stove. "I hated every minute of it, listening to her continuous whining," said Vinny.

Vinny's defining traumatic childhood experience was his rheumatic fever, which was diagnosed when he was nine years old. Although he had felt ill for a few months prior to the actual diagnosis, his mother ignored the symptoms until one day Vinny collapsed at the entrance to his school. He was then taken by his maternal grandmother, a woman whom Vinny always felt loved by, to the "kind and brilliant German Jewish doctor who lived in the neighbourhood, named Dr E." As Vinny spoke about Dr E his eyes always welled up with tears, for this man he said, "took care of me as if I was his own son." Always gentle and supportive, always interested in what he felt and thought, and always having a solution to his painful medical situation, Dr E was viewed by Vinny as his "saviour", not just from his illness, but from his abusive parents and awful home life. Said Vinny, "That Magic Man should be made a saint before Pope John Paul II."

Although Vinny was taken very good care of by Dr E, the fact is that for about six months he was on bed rest and was home schooled (by a woman teacher whom he liked, as she often brought him butter cookies). Even worse, he was partially immobilized and had to drag himself around like a seal. That, as an adult, Vinny cannot tolerate being confined or controlled in any way makes good psychological sense. However, his primary way of coping with his illness was spending most of his time in his room watching television, listening to the radio, and reading. It was within this context, feeling alone and abandoned by his parents—he once overheard them complaining how much he was costing them in medical bills—that Vincent developed an elaborate internal life. Fuelled, in part, by such wonderful classic shows, actors, characters and books as *Sergeant Preston of the Yukon*, Charlie Chan, Jean Shepherd, *King Kong*, and such horror movies as *The Crawling Eye* and *Dracula*, and, of course, Sherlock Holmes, the latter two being his favourites, Vincent said he was able to escape into another world: "It was a comforting place where good triumphed over evil, where parents loved their children, where Christmas was celebrated by a happy family, and where the world made sense." Later, in his adult life, Vinny would sometimes comfort himself by watching one of his favourite Sherlock Holmes movies while stroking one of his favourite antique English rifles (the "rifle equals penis" analogy was, of course, pointed out by me, though Vinny didn't entirely buy it). Vinny's traumatic experience of being so ill and on bed rest actually facilitated one of the main defences he has used throughout his life, escape into fantasy, though not in the negative sense, as the term is often used. Rather, Vinny's escape into fantasy was a way of fleeing "his depression by imagining himself into the experience of another person" (Spiegelman, 2002, p. 16). Indeed, it was the redemptive nature of the imagination, what Samuel Taylor Coleridge called the "faculty vision divine" (*ibid.*, p. 20), that was the germ for the development of some of Vinny's core strivings and interests that have served him well. For example, his passion for reading: he reads five newspapers a day, he receives nearly twenty magazines a month on remarkably diverse subjects, and is perhaps the most informed person I know about a wide range of subjects. His love of beautiful things like his old guns, antiques, and hand-carved furniture, the English pub he built, history, especially English history, the three homes he owns and helped design and decorate, his devotion to his family and "family values", all can be traced back, at least in part, to those six months of being a prisoner, as he described it. Vinny, in other words, spent much of his adult life realizing in real life his idealized and idealizing childhood fantasies, with some success, I might add.

Vinny managed to survive his ordeal, even flourish at times, but it was not easy for him. In fact, one of the worst parts of it occurred after he was told he could return to his Catholic school, though he had to avoid any excessive strain on his heart. According to Vinny, what this translated to was that during recess he was literally locked in a classroom alone. In fact, there were a number of times when Vinny had to pee and did so in the garbage can. Once, he came home and his mother noticed that his underwear was stained and damp, and, he said, "She beat the hell out of me." This experience further traumatized Vinny, as can be seen in his visceral fear of being trapped, and in his intense anxiety over being kept waiting. His fear of flying is another example of this carry-over from his illness days. It has been only in the last few years that Vinny has, to some extent, mastered his flying anxiety, in part through our discussions and with some medication, and by sheer force of will, motivated mainly by his home in Europe that he loves going to with his wife.

Thus, to answer the question, "How did Vinny's problems get there?", we can say that they are a result of his dreadful upbringing.

Indeed, his personality development was distorted and disfigured through the abuse and neglect at the hands of his parents and by his debilitating childhood illness. Being narcissistically assaulted on nearly every front, it is amazing that this man has had the capacity to do as well as he has. That being said, Vinny had his serious problems when I met him: his capacity for heterosexual love was extremely truncated, his relationships with women, and, for that matter, most people, were wholly exploitative and self-aggrandizing, and he could not effectively work. In addition, he was a walking time bomb, though he was only aware of his rage and emptiness in the form of anxiety attacks and some depression, which brings us to our last question, "How do you 'fix' a guy like Vinny?"

Although I am not claiming that Vinny has been transformed into a Stradivarius, so to speak, he has made great gains in his psychoanalytically-orientated psychotherapy. For instance, he has been happily married (and faithful) to a nice woman for about ten years; he has managed to fill up his day with constructive activities and hobbies that give him and others considerable pleasure, even joy (e.g., I am thinking of the magical six-course Christmas dinner he prepares for about twenty people that takes him three days to prepare, including staying up the entire night before the actual dinner to tend to the special sauces he makes); he no longer drinks; he reports being altogether less angry at the world, and his patience has greatly increased; his racism has more or less vanished, culminating in his adopting, at the age of fifty-eight, a black African child who is being raised as a Jew (Vincent's wife is a non-practising Jew). Additionally, the word "nigger", a once frequently used word for this working-class racist, has dropped out of his vocabulary ("spics", unfortunately, is the replacement category, though even this term is used infrequently these days!). Vinny is a stay-at-home dad and loves it. Every night, when his wife comes home from work, there is a four-course gourmet dinner waiting for her, as for his older son. His original symptoms have largely vanished, and he is altogether more tolerant of the unpleasant emotions that used to drive him to drink, promiscuity, or one of his favourite pastimes, driving at 120 miles an hour while intoxicated on the open highway, bouncing off the crash barrier.

Yet, Vinny has not been a total success story. He still smokes two packs of cigarettes a day, he is obese, and he does not work (though he does not financially need to). He cannot have sexual intercourse with his wife (who does not seem to mind), though they do some kissing, foreplay, and mutual masturbation. Vinny, in other words, has not been able to integrate his purely sexual urges, which are still somewhat equated with hatred of women, ultimately his mother, with his tender, affectionate and loving feelings for his wife. As I once said to Vinny, and he agreed with my interpretation though he was not able to do much with it, emotionally speaking, he needed to find a way to integrate the two images of women he had: the sexy, though hated, whore, with the loved, though unsexy, good mother. Needless to say, I have always found it to be an irony that this man, who had sexual intercourse, usually in an alcoholic fog, with over three thousand women in a twenty-year period, could not do so with the beloved wife waiting for him in their bedroom.

What was the mechanism of change to account for Vinny's considerable progress? As with any treatment, especially a long-term one, it is hard to say. However, if I had to pinpoint one element that was most healing, it was *my* love for this man. Indeed, as Freud wrote somewhere, psychoanalysis is a "scientific cure by love". It was through my unconditional positive regard, warmth, and accurate empathy that I became something of the "good" mother that Vinny always wanted and needed. That Vinny also sensed that, like an admiring and adoring parent, I really did find him to be an extraordinary person in many ways, that I mirrored his reasonable needs and desires for affirmation, but that I had earned his respect by not letting him bully me, led *him* to fall in love with me. In other words, following Levinas, what was therapeutic about Vinny's treatment was that by my acknowledging and affirming his dignity and value, by my empathically, and in other ways, aptly responding to his neediness, and by my helping to make sense of his emotional storms, personal deficits, and internal conflicts through insightful, meaning-giving interpretations, I powerfully communicated to him that, like the good parent, I was prepared to take responsibility for him because I cherished his infinite goodness. In other words, it was my taking responsibility for the Other that ultimately transformed and healed Vinny, in part, because it potentiated in him the same capacity which rippled through his life. Love, conceived as responsibility for the Other, often before oneself, was reflected in Vinny's transformation, through moral responsibility and obligation, from a man who was mainly for himself into a being who was mainly for the Other. Although he still had strong, at times inordinate, narcissistic needs for self-affirmation, for the most part he had found more benign, "for the Other" ways to satisfy them, often requiring considerable self-sacrifice.

This move from being a selfish self to being a moral self, from ethical disablement to moral "recovery", was expressed in Vinny's changed way of being in the world: from a man who had spent nearly every waking moment "playing to the crowd", trying to maintain his "larger than life" façade, as he described it, often by manipulating others in one way or another, he became considerably less self-aggrandizing at others' expense, more capable of being "himself", of being "real"; from a man who hated women, who was incapable of relating to them except as objects to exploit sexually, he became a loving husband who often puts his wife's needs ahead of his own; from a man whose entire life was dedicated to self-serving pleasure-seeking, he became the main parental care-giver, who was lovingly and gratefully raising his adopted son; from a man who spent enormous effort trying to keep himself afloat through alcohol and reckless pleasure seeking, often putting himself and others in jeopardy, he became a sober middle-aged man satisfied with doing constructive activities that gave him and others enormous pleasure.

Conclusion

The above represents only a "short list" of some of the benefits that Vinny derived from his treatment. However, it does put into sharp focus the main thesis of this chapter, which is that good psychoanalytic psychotherapy is best conceptualized in terms of "understanding how ethical responsibility constitutes and clarifies the process of humanizing and personizing each of us through otherness" (Tallon, 2007, p. 670). To the extent that an analyst can facilitate an "upsurge of the ethical" (*ibid*., p. 664), as it did in Vinny, a patient is likely to transform himself from self-cannibalizing self-worship, towards responsibility for the Other. In a sense, like Vinny, all patients are lonely in their unrestrained, self-celebrating pseudo-autonomy and superficial sociality. Their hypertrophied narcissism reflects their isolation, estrangement, and lack of sustainable, life-justifying meaning (Williams, 2007, p. 693). It was only when Vinny's intimate relationships—first with me, through his transference and the "real" relationship, then with his oppositional teenage son, whom he had more or less "disowned", then with his wife, and, finally, with his adopted son—were lodged in a deep sense of ethical obligation to their well-being, that his relationships became more profound, more stable, and more moral (*ibid.*). Moreover, it was my "recognizing, articulating, and affirming the primordial call to care for the Other" (*ibid.*, p. 700), first in myself, then gradually in Vinny, that was healing and life-affirming for this pained man. It is precisely the skilful "therapeutic deployment of moral responsibility and purpose" (*ibid.*), in a word, love, that is the key element in the healing process.

CHAPTER EIGHT

All you need is love: on the difficulties of sustaining an adult-to-adult love relationship

"How alike are the groans of love to those of the dying"

Malcolm Lowry

One day, while I was walking to my office on Queens Boulevard, two images caught my attention. The first was a young, capped man who was walking with his girlfriend while they were engaged in lively discussion. He was holding an umbrella over her head while he got wet, if not soaked. The second image was another young man in a nasty argument with his girlfriend, culminating in his calling her a "fuckin' cunt", while she told him "fuck you, it's over, asshole". These two images, reflections of Eros (the "love instinct") and Thanatos (the "death instinct"), made me wonder about the fragile, ambivalent, and transient nature of love. That is, about "the multiple affective currents, simultaneously copresent and alternating" (Eigen, 2007, p. 747) that comprise this befuddling, at times hair-raising, but always summoning experience that we call love.

Levinas, more than most modern philosophers, has written perceptively about love, conceived as responsibility for the Other before oneself. While his altruistically-sounding descriptions are inspired and inspiring, they do not adequately take up the problems that such "for the Other" loving entails on an everyday, "real-life" basis. For most of us, it is hard enough to live according to the commandment "to love thy neighbour [i.e., significant other] as thy self". To love our significant other more than we love ourselves, to put her needs and desires before our own, let alone in a sustained manner, seems like an impossible challenge. Certainly, most of us can remember times when we acted altruistically, but such moments tend to be the exception rather than the rule. That every major religious tradition makes selfless love its ideal, the personification of what is best, most divine, is indicative of the difficulties of achieving such a mode of relatedness.

That is because to be capable of selfless, or selfless-like, love in a sustained manner requires not just the willingness to give, nurture, and comfort, it also requires the capacity to contain, if not sublimate, the opposite wishes, the "dark side" of one's make-up, the selfishness and the hostility. This, of course, is one of Freud's great insights, that the love relation is fundamentally an ambivalent one. Levinas was aware of this when he wrote about "the ambiguity of love" (1969, p. 254–255), the fact that love simultaneously involves need and desire, physicality and spirituality, immanence and transcendence, ontology and ethics. Love is impossible to pin down, to abide forever, it "ceaselessly escapes" the solicitor, it "slips away" (Levinas, 1969, p. 257). While Levinas is aware of the fragility of the love relation, his observations and descriptions are sanitized, at least to this psychoanalyst. In contrast, Germaine Greer, in *The Female Eunuch* (1972), has superbly, though harshly, captured the essence of what both Freud and, to a much lesser extent, Levinas were getting at: the difficulties, if not the impossibility, of sustaining a love relationship in real life:

> Love, love, love—all the wretched cant of it, masking egotism, lust, masochism, fantasy under a mythology of sentimental postures, of welter of self induced miseries and joys, blinding and masking the essential personalities in the frozen gestures of courtship, in the kissing and the dating and the desire, the compliments and the quarrels which vivify its barrenness. [*ibid.*, p. 72]

Of course, Greer is overstating the matter, as most people probably do not experience their spouse or significant other, their so-called love relation, as quite such hard going. That being said, and this is the central question of this chapter, what are some of the psychological impediments to achieving a more selfless mode of relatedness with one's spouse or significant other? What stands in the way of a more bountiful and generous expression of love and goodness, conceived as being responsible for the Other before oneself?

Levinas on love

In a number of revealing and thoughtful interviews (Robbins, 2001), Levinas tells us what he thinks the nature of love is, including its "essence" and its "perfection":

> 1. The responsibility for the other is the grounding moment of love. It is not really a state of mind; it is not a sentiment, but rather an obligation. The human is first of all obligation. [p. 133]
>
> 2. I think that when the other is "always other", there is the essence of love . . . The more other the other is, the more he is loved, or rather, the more he is loved, the more he is other. [p. 58]
>
> 3. To approach someone as unique to the world is to love him. Affective warmth, feeling, and goodness constitute the proper mode of this approach to the unique, the thinking of the unique. [p. 108]
>
> 4. Here in language there is the possibility of expressing in a didactic manner this paradoxical relation of love, which is not simply the fact that I know someone—it is not knowing—but the sociality irreducible to knowledge which is the essential moment of love. Practically, this goodness, this nonindifference to the death of the other, this kindness, is precisely the very perfection of love. [p. 58]

For Levinas, then, love is conceived as responsibility for the other, such that the other's being and death are more important than one's own. This, he suggests, may be "the human vocation in being" (*ibid.* p. 250). Such responsibility for the other, says Levinas, is a kind of "madness", it is "an absurd thesis" (*ibid.*, p.108). I do not know if Levinas's claim is mad or absurd, but it does seem far-fetched, if not utterly unrealistic for most people, and, for that matter, throughout history. After all, in a certain sense, as with Adam and Eve, the story of love is often a "tale of a fall from harmony into chaos and disorder" (Spiegelman, 2002, Part 1, p. 26). From Heaven to Hell via Purgatory!

How does Levinas's heady notion of love as entailing a fundamental responsibility for the Other actually play out in everyday relations between adults? To briefly answer this important question, I ask the reader to keep in mind the above list of Levinas's key terms that describe his notion of love: love is not merely a strong feeling, it is an obligation; authentic love does not mainly strive after union and fusion; it always respects the other's radical otherness and cherishes the other as unique; love is not primarily characterized by mere mutual pleasure giving and reciprocal affirmation; rather, it is expressed as acts of goodness for the sake of the other's best interests, often requiring self-sacrifice. For Levinas, there are two figures in the real world who perhaps best depict the inner attitude and outer behaviour of persons capable of living their love as responsibility for the Other: first, the devoted mother, or care-giver, second, the master teacher. The devoted mother is known through her boundless self-sacrifice, compassion, and forgiveness for her children, while the master teacher facilitates in his students the birth of a new self, a better self, a self capable of actualizing the best of its intellectual, emotional, and moral capacity. What both of these authentic figures of responsibility ideally express is that they are devoted to the other's best interests, often before their own.

All of this talk about responsibility for and to the Other, the obligation to give to the other before oneself, and the cultivation of goodness as a general existential orientation in the world, is, of course, troubling to the mainstream psychoanalyst for a number of reasons. In his view, not only is such an expectation naïve and unrealistic for most people, it flies in the face of human nature as it is usually psychoanalytically conceived: man is inherently egoistic and narcissistic, tending to put himself first, and is inclined to insensitivity and indifference to the Other. Moreover, a Levinasian approach also seems to cultivate a kind of masochistic outlook, a masochistic submission to the other's needs and desires. For the Levinasian, of course, such criticisms are questionable, for they are rooted in a set of assumptions about the human condition, one of which the Levinasian rejects: that man is originally and essentially for himself and not for the Other. We will return to the differences between the Levinasian and the Freudian outlook, and their possible conceptual and real-life synthesis, at the end of this chapter.

Two key impediments to love: narcissism and aggression

Somewhat like the great English romantic poet, Percy Bysshe Shelley, Freud depended on the notion "of Eros as the impelling spirit that rolls through all things and all human consciousness" (Spiegelman, 2002, Part 2, p. 15). Indeed, for Freud, the drive theorist, man is fundamentally pleasure seeking and lives in an erotically tinged universe. That being said, Freud and all of his subsequent followers were mainly concerned with what gets in the way of the wide and deep expression of Eros. That is, Eros defined more broadly than simply as the sexual instincts, but rather as a poetic metaphor for the life-affirming life force. While this subject could be the basis of another twenty-four volumes of Freud's *Standard Edition*, I wish to focus on two key impediments to the proper expression of Eros, which are inordinate narcissism, or what is commonly called selfishness, and aggression, or what is commonly called hostility. Indeed, Melanie Klein, one of Freud's great disciples, the originator of object-relations theory, noted that the main human struggle is "between love and hate, between care and concern for others and their malicious destruction" (Alford, 1998, p. 120). Let's take a closer look at these two impediments to Eros, first narcissism, though as will become clear, they are often, if not always, interconnected, if not mingled.

Narcissism

Levinas, like Freud, assumed that man is fundamentally egotistical. Man takes his own needs and desires as most important, and, in most instances, he thinks about the other person second. In our culture, and for that matter in most of the cultures I am aware of, human beings seem to be originally, and mainly, for themselves, and not for the Other (though altruism and other pro-social sentiments are not uncommon). Altruistic behaviour, even everyday kindness, like someone holding the door open for you, is so striking because it is rare. In a simple gesture of courtesy, the other's respect and dignity is decisively affirmed.

Why are people typically so self-centred and selfish? In a word, following the Buddha, it is due to the "three poisons": greed, hatred, and delusion (greedy delusional hatred being perhaps the most toxic mix). In psychoanalytic terminology, greed mainly refers to the wish to aggressively possess all the goodness of the other; hatred refers to the persistent wish to injure or destroy the despised other; and delusion refers to holding to a false or unchallengeable conviction about the other, and/or about how the world holds together. To the extent that these "poisons", these affect/thought clusters, are not modulated, transformed, or eliminated, one is likely to be self-centred and selfish, and, of course, hostile in outlook and behaviour. As I have shown in the previous chapter on psychotherapy in general, the main reason, at least beyond the basic human inclination to being absorbed in the three poisons and their derivatives, is early inadequate parenting and other harmful-to-the-self childhood experiences. Such experiences force the person to circle the wagons, as it were, and to assume an inordinate self-protective and self-referential mode of being in the world. Within the context of an intimate relation, often this mode of being has a psychologically "violent" feel to it, both in its active mode, that is, in its aggressive and even mean-spirited expression, and in its passive mode, in its emotional withdrawing and other forms of passive aggression.

For example, in greed, as Greenberg and Mitchell point out (1983, pp. 128–129), the needy and dependent person wants to obtain all the contents, the love and nurturance, of the good other, regardless of its impact on the other. Like the farmer in Aesop's famous fable of "The Goose Who Laid the Golden Eggs", it is irrelevant what terrible harm can befall the other as a result of his greed: "Thinking to get all the gold that the goose could give in one go, he killed it, and opened it only to find—nothing." That is, most often, the greedy person experiences the other's nurturance and goodness as inadequate and begrudges, if not greatly resents, his control over it. For instance, the husband who wants his non-working wife to tend to him, have dinner waiting for him after a hard day's work, and then gets furious when she does not, for no good reason in his view, he is reacting like an entitled infant who expects his mother to nurture him on demand, to be perfect. In the mind of the regressed husband, his wife becomes all "bad", with what he takes to be her withholding behaviour reflecting her selfish and hoarding nature, the basis for his fury.

In hatred, as Rycroft has pointed out (1968, p. 61), the person has a sustained wish to harm or kill the hated other (in contrast to anger, which is a passing feeling towards someone one cares about or loves). As Lord Byron wrote in his famous poem *Don Juan*, "Now hatred is by far the longest pleasure; Men love in haste, but they detest at leisure". Whether the wish to do harm is directed at a hated or loved other, whether it is a sustained or transient wish, according to Freud, hate is most often a response to threats to the ego's stability and integrity, though in his later writings he viewed it as an expression of the death instinct. In other words, in general, most forms of hatred, especially as they play out in ordinary love relations, are a response to frustration and conflict pertaining to one's narcissistic needs to be respected, valued, and loved. Most often however, these needs are inordinate and produce hatred in the aggrieved person, who more or less experiences his significant other as unreasonably, if not arbitrarily, depriving. So, for example, a needy and dependent woman who experiences her husband as distracted and fundamentally ungratifying of her need to be cherished, may develop a deep sense of resentment of him, leading to endless skirmishes and more serious relationship problems.

Finally, we come to delusion, a persistent false belief held in the face of strong contradictory evidence. Delusion is a more subtly acting poison, at least as it plays out in intimate relationships. There are many common delusions, or delusion-like views that people hold to in their love relationships. For example, the man who believes that his wife should be all things to him all the time, that she should always be perky and happy, his antidepressant as it were, is expecting something that is not reasonable from his wife. As I have noted elsewhere (2003, pp. 142–143), for St Augustine, each object of love fits with the inner disposition and expectations of the lover and it is a mistake to expect more from a particular object of love than its unique nature can provide. Such "disordered love", as Augustine called it, that is, expecting more from an object of love than it is capable of providing, is usually anxiety-ridden, frightened, greedy, and clinging. In contrast, "rightly ordered love" allows us to evaluate things according to their proper value and priority; it helps us to generate reasonable and appropriate goals, desires, and actions for the pursuit of, and relationship to, what we love.

Quite simply, the goal of analysis, at least in part, is to transform in the broadest way possible, greed into generosity, hatred into loving-kindness, and delusion into realistic thinking, that is, viewing things in terms of their "true" nature. To accomplish this is, of course, no easy task, for it requires the transformation of the substructure that supports this self- and other-destructive mode of being in the world—the prison-house of the selfish-self. That is, it requires the subversion of one's narcissistic identification with one's unreasonable desires, the irrational, often child-based, feelings and thoughts that we are utterly bound to, that constitute the "I", that tend to subvert proper ego functioning, and pollute the very core, so to speak, of the person himself. In other words, only when one has overcome, or at least modulated, one's selfish cravings (infantile narcissism, in psychoanalytic parlance) by reconfiguring one's subjectivity along less self-centred and self-interested lines, can the main impediments to love, at least as Levinas conceives it, be overcome. One of the main difficulties with accomplishing such a reconfiguring of one's subjectivity, from mainly self- to other-regarding, is the second great impediment to love: the problem of aggression, that is, the irrational, self-subverting human propensity to hurting those we love.

Aggression

As one gets older, it becomes increasingly apparent just how limited, flawed, and downright deficient one's behaviour is in one's love relation. Following Freud, we can say that most, if not all, people "are born with limited capacities to pursue the good, and left to our own devices all of us will betray ourselves and our fellow man" (Pattison, 1988, p. 89). Nietzsche, a precursor of Freud in many ways, and someone the young Freud greatly admired, put the matter more severely by describing man as "the cruelest of animals" (Assoun, 2002, p. 151). Thus, it is not altogether surprising that human relationships are often infiltrated by man's "dark side", by the "three poisons" and other forms of destructive emotions, thoughts and, most importantly, behaviour. Put straightforwardly, we are all fundamentally flawed beings, often inclined to being selfish, impatient, dishonest, envious, mean-spirited, and even cruel in our relationships, including our primary adult love relation.

That being said, there is one aspect of human aggression as expressed within love relations that I want to elaborate further, which is the fact that, almost always, the aggression directed at one's significant other reflects the perpetrator's belief, or at least wish, that the other person be what he wants her to be. We all suffer, at least to some extent, from what, in the surgeon's world of elective plastic surgery, is called the Pygmalion Complex, the zealous, if not obsessive wish to make beautiful and perfect people, according to what we think they should be. This belief or wish, actually more a demand, is rooted in an inflated infantile narcissism, a kind of hypertrophied pride, that unashamedly asserts that the universe, including one's significant other, is not fashioned as it should be, that is, as one wants it to be, and, therefore, the significant other must be reconfigured, with oneself as God, the Creator. In other words, in this view, deployment of aggression in most forms, at least in the most rudimentary sense, boldly expresses the narcissistic claim that one is essentially self-sufficient, self-sustaining, and self-dependent, and that one does not need anyone or anything, except to the extent that one can use the other to feed one's infantile, pleasure-seeking, self-aggrandizing desires. Put simply, within the context of intimate relationships, aggression is almost always a way of "strong-arming" the other, experienced as a satellite in one's orbit, to affirm the perpetrator's narcissistic grandiose self that imagines itself as a self-dependent Creator. Aggression is, thus, a form of self-valorization and self-glorification; it is an aggressive selfishness (Assoun, 2000, pp. xxxiv, 61)

Thus, we can say that one of the goals of analysis is a kind of re-education of moral identity (*ibid.*, p. xxxviii). That is, transforming moral being, in psychoanalytic terms, sublimating one's primitive, destructive narcissism/aggression into more "for the Other" ways of being in the world. In this view, following Levinas, sublimation, one of the hallmarks of any "successful" analysis, is conceived as a fundamentally ethical process, the channelling of selfish and hostile impulses and energies into activities regarded as more socially acceptable, that is, for the Other, most broadly conceived.

Levinas vs. *Freud on love*

As the reader must sense by now, my two intellectual lights, Levinas and Freud, have rather different views, or at least different emphases, about what constitutes adult-to-adult love, and, perhaps more importantly, what is actually possible, especially in a sustained manner, between two people who reside in what they call a love relation. Let's take a closer look at Levinas and Freud on the problem of love, and see if there is a way of bridging their seemingly divergent views, so that we have a possibly workable formulation that can be helpful to *real* people in *real* love relationships. It is precisely such a dialectical formulation, where love is viewed as a welding of opposites, perhaps best personified in the love–death theme mentioned earlier, that I put forward at the conclusion of this chapter. Such a view reflects Freud's "paradoxical proposition", as he called it, "that the normal man is not only far more immoral than he believes but also far more moral than he knows . . ." (Freud, 1923b, p. 52).

Levinas's conception of love, quoted earlier, "The responsibility for the other is the grounding moment of love . . . when the other is 'always other', there is the essence of love . . .", rests on an assumption about the human condition that is at odds with Freud. "I speak of responsibility as the essential, primary and fundamental structure of subjectivity" (Levinas, 1985, p. 95). In other words, according to Levinas, we are "hard-wired" to be responsible for the Other. As I have pointed out elsewhere, for the psychoanalyst such a view sounds implausible (Marcus, 2008). Indeed, Levinas does not really tell us that he "knows for sure" how to effectively substantiate his bold claim. This lack of adequate substantiation, or at least clarification, is noteworthy, especially when we appreciate a crucial feature of language: meaning is not fixed, but is emergent, tied to specific situations and constantly changing. Thus, the concept of responsibility, like any concept or term, cannot itself convey to us how it is to be properly used. There is no set of rules or instructions that intrinsically comes with the concept; it is open-ended and revisable. Therefore, if the proper usage of a term or concept like responsibility is simply the usage communally judged to be proper, and is no more predetermined than idiosyncratic individual usage, then the "essential, primary and fundamental" nature of responsibility is questionable, ethically troubling. Put more starkly, if the meaning of language is really no more stable than the particular situations it may be used to describe, then one could conceivably claim that the Nazis were acting in a manner that reflected "responsibility for the Other" in killing the Jews, who were destroying the Aryan nation. That the concept of responsibility for the Other is radically philosophical, without a fixed ethical meaning, and therefore open to abuse, is not, so far as I know, considered by Levinas.

A second psychoanalytically-orientated criticism of Levinas's claim that "responsibility for the Other is an essential, primary and fundamental structure of subjectivity" is that the notion of the other is not something that we come into the world with (Marcus, 2008, p. 45). So far as we know, the infant only apprehends or "knows" that there is an "other" well after birth. Therefore, to speak of "responsibility for the Other" as, in a sense, hard-wired, does not take into consideration that the infant's sense of the "other" is a later developmental acquisition. Even more troubling is the fact that an infant's notion of "responsibility", as conventionally understood, and certainly in a Levinasian ethical sense, is an even later developmental acquisition. All of this raises the question of whether it is reasonable to claim that "responsibility for the Other" can be described as an essential, primary, and fundamental structure of subjectivity.

Although such criticisms of Levinas are not easily or convincingly answered, the fact is that Levinas is correctly capturing a dimension of the adult-to-adult love experience, at least in its ideal form: "responsibility for the other is the grounding moment of love", but only its grounding moment, not its sum and substance in everyday reality. There is a real–ideal dichotomy that Levinas's description of love does not adequately address, let alone resolve. For most people do not seem to relate to their significant Other, at least in a sustained way, the way Levinas describes love. The "I" of the mature person will recognize such a conception as a valid ideal, but not an easily reachable goal, to put it mildly. As Sartre said, every book is an attempt to improve one's biography, and one wonders if Levinas's idealistic descriptions of love reflect the way he would wish love relationships to be, rather than the way they usually play out in real life. Love relations, like all human relationships are messy and complicated, laced with contradictory feelings and attitudes, as Freud has noted, and as most honest and self-aware people, at least in Western society, will tell you.

In contrast to Levinas, Freud's view of love is driven, if not limited, by his guiding assumption about the human condition, that man is fundamentally egotistical and pleasure seeking. For Freud (Marcus, 2008, p. 105), love is conceptualized from his instinctivist perspective in which Eros, Freud's gracefully expressive metaphor for the life force and sexual instincts, though concretely manifested as sexual satisfaction, is the core of what is meant by love. In this view, all forms of love, including in their sublimated expressions, as, for example, in love of God, music, an idea, or one's dog, are construed as derivatives of instinct and their main purpose is to give instinctual gratification. In a sense, then, for Freud, since love has a libidinous source, that is, it emanates from the instinctual wellspring that constitutes the human condition, all love is essentially love of a need-satisfying object. So-called normal or mature love, says Freud in his *Three Essays on the Theory of Sexuality* (1905d), comes about from the amalgamation of kind-hearted, adoring and sexual feelings towards a person of the opposite sex ("significant other", we would say these days). In contrast to mature love, neurotic love does not adequately acknowledge, let alone affirm the separateness of the other, that is, his unique individuality (e.g., his special characteristics, capacities, and potentialities), that which makes him different from oneself. Moreover, in neurotic love, the neurotic requires frequent and pronounced validating and affirming responses from his or her significant other, and tends to get very anxious, angry, and/or depressed, or all three, when it is not forthcoming. In addition, for Freud, mature love requires object constancy—"integration of originally separate, unconscious mental representations of 'good' and 'bad' objects into more realistic and stable representations combining the 'good' and 'bad' qualities" (Person, Cooper, & Gabbard, 2005, p. 555). This capacity to sustain a lasting and reasonable relationship with a specific, single, separate other obviously requires a well-developed sense of autonomy and integration (e.g., a good sense of self-cohesion, self-continuity, and self-esteem, among other elements). In short, for Freud, love is marked by genital primacy in sexuality (i.e., reaching the genital level, the final phase of libidinal development), and object love in relationships with others (i.e., love that discerns and values the other's otherness). "Loving and being loved", the "union of mental and bodily satisfaction", says Freud (1930a, p. 82), is perhaps the best way for achieving "a positive fulfilment of happiness" (Freud, 1915a, p. 169) in one's life.

Finally, for Freud, what more or less determines the nature of the love relationship, its formation, structuring, and the "feel" to it, is one's earliest experiences with one's care-givers. That is, love has, as its paradigm, the earliest exclusive attachment with the care-giving parent. Thus, as Freud famously said, all love relations are a "refinding of the object"; that is, our choice of a love partner mainly represents a fixation on one's parents, what Freud called transference love in the analytic context. For Freud, what constitutes the difference between ordinary love in "real life" and transference love in the analytic context is a question of degree. Love's "irrationality, its compulsiveness, its frequently self-damaging aspects", says Fine (1979, p. 48), are best comprehended in terms of the adult's imperfect relationship with his care-givers.

Thus, we have two formulations of the nature of love: for Levinas, love is responsibility for the Other before oneself, whereas for Freud, love is the love of a need-satisfying object (i.e., significant other). Is there a way of bringing together these two valid, but incomplete, divergent views of love? In particular, how can Freud's, in my view, truer-to-real-life description of love as essentially ambivalent be joined with Levinas's ideal-sounding "for the Other" formulation?

"Moment love"—love conceived as a dialectical tension

The capacity for what is termed mature adult-to-adult love depends on a number of factors as described above, perhaps the most important being the ability to "manage" one's ambivalence, ambivalence broadly described. Love requires the mingling or balancing of opposites, for example, the reasonable needs and desires of the self *vs.* those of the Other, closeness *vs.* distance, dependence *vs.*

independence, and, of course, affection *vs.* hostility. The latter opposites are the sharpest expression of ambivalence, a derivative of the love–death struggle that underlies all the love relations mentioned earlier. Exactly how most people accomplish the integration, or at least reasonable balancing of the such opposites, and these are only a few of them, is not exactly clear, though no progression in a love relation is likely to occur without doing so. Put simply, unless one can live within the dialectical tension between Eros and Thanatos, ideally with a tilting towards the positive side of the ambivalence, towards Eros, one is not going to be able to adequately sustain a love relation with a significant Other.

If love is potentially so redeeming, if it is so utterly self-, other- and life-affirming, at least as most of us construe it at its best, why then must love be a "moment love" when love and the redemptive vision of love are present, though interspersed with times when the difficult, if not hellish aspects of the love relation dominate (Greenberg, 1977, pp. 33)? In other words, how does one keep the redemptive vision of love alive and present in the face of its death-tinged opposite?

The answer, or at least an important aspect of the answer, is to learn how to reside in what William Wordsworth called the "border states", the space between love and death. This imaginary place, the boundary between two people, I call "moment love/moment death" is best known by its experienced paradoxes (Carnes, 1989, p. 245). For example, "fidelity to oneself" leads to being faithful to the Other; recognizing and admitting personal limitations and faults creates a deeper understanding and acceptance of the Other's limits and inadequacies; honesty with oneself fosters greater realism with the Other; to be reasonably loving of oneself liberates new caring capacities that can be utilized for the best interests of the Other; to nurture oneself creates new resources of support for the Other. And, of course, to do all of these things encourages the significant other to be "forgiving, realistic, honest, loving, and nurturing" in return. While, for Levinas, being for the Other should not be based on the expectation of reciprocity, as then it is fundamentally self-love, the fact is that most love relations, at least most of the time in the practical realm, probably operate according to the norm of reciprocity, that is, they tend to be symmetrical—"I do for you, you do for me"—and not, as Levinas wants, asymmetrical, that is, selfless. This is where Levinas and Freud disagree, and from my clinical and life experience, Freud, sadly, seems to be more accurate than Levinas, at least pertaining to our current era. Most of us are not saints, not even nearly so, as our love is fundamentally selfish, not selfless. This is not as bad as it sounds, because the "right" behaviour—acting lovingly though for the "wrong" reason, narcissistic gratification—is still a lot better than acting unlovingly. Indeed, from a psychoanalytic point of view, all selfless-like acts have some kind of narcissistic "pay-off", though the predominant motivation—being for oneself *vs.* being for the Other—is an important difference in terms of individual psychology. In a certain sense, in a love relation what most counts is behaviour, not motivation, or, as the saying goes, "faking it is making it"!

If one were to identify three interrelated, essential elements in a high-functioning adult- to-adult love relation, elements that must animate the imaginary border space of "moment love/moment death", so that the death-tinged forces do not overwhelm and destroy workable love, I would say that hope, faith, and forgiveness are extremely important. Some brief elaboration of these three key interrelated elements, elements that have been under-researched in the psychological literature, is a fitting way to conclude this chapter.

The redemptive triad: hope, faith, and forgiveness

Although Levinas's claim that "responsibility for the Other is the grounding moment of love" is certainly plausible, the fact is that, for responsibility to survive and flourish, it, too, often needs to be "grounded" in something else, or be fuelled by something else, equally, if not more, personally summoning. That is, perhaps the best defence against ambivalence in a love relation, the potentially relationship-destroying dichotomies, contradictions, and incongruities, the ever-present shadow of Thanatos, is a mindfully held counter-vision, a new way of thinking, imagining, and valuing the Other. This counter-vision is, in part, characterized by infinite hope, "a passion for what is possible", as Kierkegaard described it, faith, an attitude of openness, especially to the truth, fused with absolute trust and, finally, perhaps the ultimate expression of love and reparation, forgiveness, the capacity for pardoning the significant other for a mistake or wrongdoing directed towards oneself.

As Levinas noted, "The other is . . . the first rational teaching, the condition of all teaching" (Levinas, 1969, pp. 171). Wiesel has aptly rendered one of the important meanings of Levinas's hard-to-understand claim that the Other is the teacher, as it relates to the psychology of hope within a love relationship: "just as despair can come to one only from other human beings, hope, too, can be given only by other human beings". Hope, that necessary sense of destination to somewhere better, the space between dreams and reality, that imaginative victory over experience, is a kind of unrefuseable obligation if a love relationship is to endure. Moreover, paradoxically, hope is also the reward for one's faith in the Other, in the Other's infinite goodness. Erikson has aptly made a similar point in describing hope as the essential "ego virtue" that emerges after a successful negotiation of the psychosocial stage of infancy he calls "basic trust versus basic mistrust." Says Erikson, hope "is the enduring belief in the attainability of fervent wishes, in spite of the dark urges and rages which mark the beginning of existence" (1964, p. 118). Moreover, continues Erikson, as hope is cultivated by the parents deep and abiding faith that what the child does has significance and is "good", the child's overall feeling of hopefulness will eventually be transformed into grown-up faith, a self-assurance that does not require either evidence or reason that the universe is essentially trustworthy and benign (*ibid.*, p. 153). In other words, within a love relation, the lover ideally has a deeply internalized sense of hope and its mature derivative faith that helps animate, if not sustain, the relationship, especially during hard times. Moreover, as Erich Fromm has noted, while hope means to be prepared at every moment for that which is not yet born, it also means not becoming frantic if there is no birth during the course of one's love relation.

> To love means to commit oneself without guarantee, to give oneself completely in the hope that our love will produce love in the loved person. Love is an act of faith, and whoever is of little faith is also of little love. [Fromm, 1956, pp. 127–128]

Faith, like its cousin hope, pertains to things not actually seen between two people, "a passionate intuition", as Wordsworth described it. Similar to hope, faith often tends to originate, or, at least, is most sharply perceived, in the darkness. It is often a response to difficulties in a relationship. Indeed, as Heschel noted (1955, pp. 132, 155), the essence of faith is faithfulness to a moment, fidelity to a self- and Other-consecrating event, to a transforming response between two people that reveals the awesome, mysterious, ineffable goodness of the Other, the basis for trust in the future. Such a faith gives one the strength of waiting, the patient acceptance of the Other's concealment of his goodness, especially when relationships are rough going. Faith, in other words, evokes a sense of daring confidence that love is stronger than death, what in religious circles is called God's grace. As religious scholar Smith wrote (1979), faith reflects the human tendency "to see, to feel, to act in terms of a transcendent dimension", to sense meaning and significance that is more than simply ordinary and commonplace. Faith is vital to maintaining a love relationship and living, for it provides it with "coherence and direction", it connects one to "shared trusts and loyalties", it existentially "grounds" one's "personal stances and loyalties in a sense of relatedness to a larger frame of reference", and it helps people to cope adequately with the "limit conditions" and inevitable suffering of existence, all this by using compelling psychological and other resources that have a sense of "ultimacy" and transcendence (Shafranske, 1996, p. 168).

Finally, we come to forgiveness, the pardoning of the Other's misdeeds when one feels mistreated, if not victimized. Indeed, as the well-known saying goes, there is no love without forgiveness and no forgiveness without love. Forgiveness expresses the renewal of hope that is essential to any workable love relation. Indeed, in a love relation we all periodically feel hard done by, that is, narcissistically assaulted, or at least disrespected in terms of what we think we should be getting from our significant other: greater care, more accurate empathy, willingness to sacrifice, and the like. Such narcissistic assaults tend to foster the resentment, anger, revenge, and other forms of aggression that are so common in intimate relationships in one form or another. However, the capacity to forgive, the compassionate reconfiguration of thought and feeling about the other that forgiveness requires, generates a new moral context for the interpretation of the other's hurtful behaviour. When the aggrieved person chooses to give up *his* resentment, even hate of the perpetrator for his misdeed, that signifies that he is, in effect, willing to deal with the pain that underlies the narcissistic rage evoked by his significant other's misdeed. In other words, forgiveness increases one's range of alternatives just as it enhances one's freedom to grow and develop. It is the basis for the healing process that needs to occur to keep a love relation from disintegrating as a result of our all too human capacity to be intentionally and/or unintentionally destructive to our loved Other. As Voltaire said, "every man is guilty of all the good he didn't do".

"All you need is love", says the famous Beatle song. This is a simple but compelling truth; however, as I hope I have shown, sustaining a love relation, let alone one that is mainly "for the Other", such as Levinas has in mind, is no easy accomplishment. For living and loving according to a regulative principle of "responsibility for the Other", of being for the Other before oneself, requires considerable modulation and sublimation of the human tendency to be inordinately narcissistic and aggressive, that is, aggressively selfish. Moreover, love requires the development of the mature capacity for hope, faith, and forgiveness, these being necessary to support the love relation, a relation that is always fragile, given the ubiquity of ambivalence. For love to flourish, one must adequately negotiate the dialectical tension of "love–death", to give up the controlling fantasy/demand, that there is anything more than "moment love/moment death". As F. Scott Fitzgerald wrote, "the test of a first rate intelligence is the ability to hold two opposed ideas in mind at the same time and still retain the ability to function. One should, for example, be able to see that things are hopeless and yet be determined to make them otherwise."

This view of adult-to-adult love relations may strike the reader as unduly pessimistic, but one should take some comfort in the words of the great American Protestant theologian, Niebuhr, words that remind us that, while sustaining a love relation has its enormous difficulties, it also is the answer to our ultimate questions and, even better, it is an eternally renewable resource for those who have the necessary self-understanding and self-mastery:

> Nothing worth doing is completed in our lifetime.
> Therefore, we are saved by hope.

Nothing true or beautiful or good makes complete sense in any immediate context of history. Therefore, we are saved by faith.

Nothing we do, however virtuous, can be accomplished alone. Therefore, we are saved by love.

No virtuous act is quite as virtuous from the standpoint of our friend or foe as from our own. Therefore, we are saved by the final form of love which is forgiveness. [http://www.brainyquote.com/quotes/authors/r/reinhold_niebuhr.html]

CHAPTER NINE

Looking for God in all the right places: on developing an "adult" religious outlook

> "If I want to fix my mind on what I mean by absolute or ethical value . . . one particular experience presents itself to me . . . I believe the best way of describing it is to say that when I have it *I wonder at the existence of the world* . . . It is the experience of seeing the world as a miracle"
>
> Ludwig Wittgenstein

In a certain sense, we are all spiritual wanderers, that is, we are all on a journey of self-discovery in one form or another. For some, like Freud, such a journey leads to a mainly secular conclusion; for others, like Levinas, the voyage of self-discovery leads to a mainly religious outlook, though not necessarily one that is correlated with institutional religion or familiar notions of spirituality. That being said, the inner journey and its conclusion is usually not so straightforward, but has many swings and roundabouts. For example, although Freud was an atheist, he did acknowledge, especially as he got older, the positive value of monotheistic religion, Judaism in particular. According to Edmundson, author of *The Death of Sigmund Freud: The Legacy of His Last Days*, Freud believed that

> taking God into the mind enriches the individual immeasurably. The ability to believe in an internal, invisible God vastly improves people's capacity for abstraction . . . the belief in an unseen God may prepare the ground not only for science and literature and law but also for intense introspection. [Edmundson, 2007, p. 17]

Levinas, while a practising Orthodox Jew (though a heterodox one), had a view of religion that was hardly conventional, and in many ways it was critical of the monotheistic religion many of us in the Western world have been raised on in one form or another: God was not a "strange magician", or "lesser demon", "a fairly primary sort of God" who "dished out prizes, inflicted punishment or pardoned sins—a God who, in His goodness, treated men like children". Rather, an "adult's God", Levinas claims, reveals Himself "precisely through the void of the child's heaven. This is the moment when God retires from the world and hides His face" (1990a, p. 143).

As the above quotations suggest, "God talk" is almost always a dicey matter, not only because of its complexity and ambiguity, but also because most people "discover" God, or at least originally learn about God, through their childhood familial, communal, and educational experiences, and, therefore, often hold those views—and the unconscious sensibility that goes along with them—dearly and tenaciously. On this point Freud was right, belief in God and the way one "does" religion, is often consciously and unconsciously tied to how one feels and thinks about one's parents or early caregivers, family, and faith community.

In this chapter, mainly drawing from Levinas and Freud, I want to describe some of the elements that constitute a so-called "adult" religious outlook, a way of being in the world in which, among other characteristics, "man transcends his individual ego" and "transfers the center of reference to others, and thus transforms self-love into, simply, love" for the Other, broadly described (Abrams, 1971, p. 296). What I am calling an "adult" religious outlook is, in part, achieved and expressed through one's mode of relatedness to God, through the imagination, via creative visualization, through nature, via the visual experience of beauty, and, perhaps most importantly, through the Other, via responsibility. My claim is that, regardless of which religious tradition one is lodged in, an "adult" life-affirming way of being religious (or spiritual, as some call it) usually involves, in one form or another, the capacity to fully engage God, Nature, and the Other, in their luminous otherness, such being the surest way to the higher level of integration, unity, and being that is correlated with paradise here on earth. Indeed, to achieve what Schelling called "eternity within himself", an "inner identity with the Absolute" (*ibid.*, p. 356), or any other similar formulation that believers use to express their loving and serene connection to God (or its equivalent in Eastern religions), requires a dangerous "quest through the uncharted regions of our own mind" (*ibid.*, p. 285). As Confucius noted, "the mind of man is more perilous than mountains or rivers, harder to understand than Heaven". There are, as we shall see, many psychological tendencies that impede one's capacity to fully engage God, Nature, and the Other, to dwell in the eternal dimension of your being and, thereby, achieve the transformation of consciousness that often leads to the "experiential paradise", what Rousseau called "the supreme felicity" (*ibid*, pp. 347, 385), that, in psychoanalytic terms, is equated with greater autonomy, personality integration, and, perhaps most importantly, peace of mind.

Playing "hide and seek" with God

The saintly Mother Teresa shocked the world, especially the religious world, when she wrote in her missionary letters that amid the suffering masses that she so selflessly and ably tended to, she failed to feel "even the smallest glimmer" of God's presence in the world. "I am told that God lives in me," she noted, "and yet the reality of darkness and coldness and emptiness is so great that nothing touched my soul." Furthermore, while greatly upset by the suffering she witnessed, Mother Teresa longed for God "with all power of my soul—and yet between us there is terrible separation". "Jesus", she wrote, "is the absent one . . . I don't have Him" (*The Week*, 2007b, p. 19).

This is a powerful testimonial, coming from a woman depicting the best of Christian faith and sacrificial activism, and yet her reflections, quoted above, disruptive as they are, put into sharp focus a problem that most honest spiritual wanderers and God-seekers struggle with: how can one engage God, however he is consciously, cognitively conceived, to cleave to Him in a sustained manner as a real-life transformative force, one that altogether enhances us as humans while making us better people, more capable of loving and serving the Other—human and otherwise—in the deepest and broadest way possible?

While such a complex and compelling question has been "kicked around" for centuries among the great religious traditions, and still is (Marcus, 2003), I want to focus on one neglected aspect, at least in the psychoanalytic and psychological literature, of man's search for God, which is that it requires a powerful imagination, among other internal capacities, to believe in, or even transiently apprehend God, let alone rigorously live a God-animated life that affirms the Good, the Beautiful, and the True. By imagination, I mean, following the great English Romantic poets, the capacity to form images and ideas in the mind, especially of things never seen or never directly experienced, which, nevertheless, have a life-affirming significance, especially in matters that are typically of ultimate importance to most people. I am suggesting that "heaven, hell and paradise are not outward places but states of mind", that "imagination" signifies "the faculty of vision and eternal truth" (*ibid.*, p. 54). Thus, it is a crucial resource for developing a more ethically self-enhancing, "for the Other" way of being in the world. Shelley perceptively emphasized this important point when he wrote that "the great instrument of the moral good is the Imagination". The imagination helps us discover deeper truths about ourselves and the world, truths that are ethically deepening, just as they are beautiful.

It is certainly true that people come to God from many different motivations and by many different trajectories, some reasonable and wholesome, and some utterly unreasonable and detrimental, both to themselves and to others. With regard to the latter group, one just has to think of the religious person whose God is mainly characterized by "fire and brimstone", and whose devotion to Him and to His Laws is largely driven by neurotic guilt and a fear of punishment. Such judgemental people drive themselves and those around them crazy, for they make life unbearably restricted and tormented, almost completely discouraging most kinds of normative, responsible pleasure seeking. In other words, for such fundamentalist types, seeking pleasure in life is like licking honey off a razor blade. Other perverse religious types include those who think they have found the Absolute Truth about God and are willing to murder others, non-believers and the like, justifying killing those who live life differently in the name of serving Him.

While there have been tons of books and scholarly articles written about both of these two religious types, what interests me in this concluding chapter is the way the average thoughtful, spiritually-inclined person can better access his or her God in a way that is more life-enhancing for both oneself, for those one loves, and for the larger community. It should be noted, at the outset of this chapter, that I am not weighing in on the heady, if not unanswerable question of whether there is or is not a God, whether the existence of a God can be proved. Rather, my focus is on how people work positively with God, as it were, constructively "use" Him in their lives, as I have observed in my work with the Jewish, Christian, Muslim, Hindu, and Buddhist patients whom I have seen in psychotherapy and child custody evaluations over the years in the most ethnically diverse borough in New York City, or, for that matter, in the USA: Queens. My own struggles with God, religion, and spirituality are, of course, also relevant here.

As I have already insinuated, one of the key ways of being able to engage God as a living presence, or at least the one way that I think needs to be better appreciated, is the power of the imagination to infuse "the infinite into the finite", the eternal into the temporal. Following Blake, according to this view, reality is fundamentally spiritual, and it is through the imagination that one can perceive it as such: "Imagination is a spiritual sensation", it is undoubtedly the "first principle" of knowledge, and all others spring from it (Preminger, 1965, pp. 373–375). As Einstein noted, "imagination is more important than knowledge. Knowledge is limited, imagination encircles the world". Thus, imagination can be thought of as a kind of "spiritual optics". Without the capacity for imaginative vision, it is nearly impossible to perceive, let alone experience, the wonder, beauty, and goodness of life. As Keats said, "I am certain of nothing but the holiness of the heart's affections, and the truth of the imagination".

How does the imagination bring God alive, make Him and our relationship to Him a life-affirming, life-enhancing force in our lives, one that brings us, following Levinas, closer to goodness, the ultimate basis of what constitutes the Good Life?

Drawing mainly from the late Irish poet, philosopher, and Catholic scholar, John O'Donohue (2004), I will now briefly describe some important ways that the imagination can be used to access God, not in a mechanical, reductive, or simplistic manner, but rather as a sensibility, as a capacity to perceive and feel, to respond aesthetically and emotionally to God, however momentarily or vague it may be for some. My claim is that unless one has developed the deep inner capacity to imagine, one will be, for the most part, deprived of access to the living God, whether God is mainly conceived as a superordinate, pristine philosophical idea and/or redemptive personal concept, the experience of beauty through Nature, or selfless service to the Other. In actuality, God/Nature/Other are best psychologically conceptualized as one, as inextricably linked metaphors for signifying different aspects of the longing for the "paradisal unity of being" (Abrams, 1971, p. 237). It is a search for that seamless fluency of being that we had when we were unselfconscious children utterly in love with the world, and that we glimpse when we imaginatively, respectfully, and wholeheartedly engage the mysterious, luminous, otherness of God, Nature, and the Other.

The imagination, says O'Donohue, brings "wonderful gifts" to those who mindfully nurture and use it, including accessing the beauty, truth and goodness of God. The poet W. H. Auden felt similarly when he wrote that for the romantic poet the "imagination is a power of vision which enables man to perceive the sacred truth behind sensory phenomena and therefore the noblest of all mental faculties" (1966, p. ix). For example, the imagination is "like a lantern" that illuminates new "inner landscapes" and "regions of the mind" that help create an openness to the transcendent that allows one possibly to glimpse and sense God's presence. For the person with an "adult" religious outlook, as I have called it, God is more clearly perceived and strongly felt because his mind is not dulled and his heart is not blunted; in psychoanalytic language, such a person is not trapped in the endless thicket of neurosis, including rigidly relating only to surface reality. Rather, he "engages the world visually in an imaginative way", and, thus, he notices new things around him that are manifestations of the divine, of divine warmth and caring, as he interprets them. The Jewish philosopher,

Heschel, called this the experience of "wonder", of "radical amazement" (1955, p. 47) and he noted, correctly I think, that the "indifference to the sublime wonder of living is the root of sin" (*ibid.*, p. 43). My point is beautifully and succinctly captured by the words of the German poet and satirist Heinrich Heine, who observed that "the grandeur of the universe is commensurate with the soul that surveys it". This means that God can be engaged if one uses one's God-given capacity to imagine, as Levinas says, "something other than being, beyond being". God, so mysteriously conceived, continues a befuddling Levinas as he tries to find the right words, or the almost right words, to evoke his notion of God, "is not simply the 'first other', or the 'other *par excellence*', or the 'absolutely other', but other than the other, other otherwise" (1998c, p. 69). Needless to say, imagining such a God requires an extremely capacious imagination! However, I think Levinas is pointing to a critical need, especially for those who have been touched by the sceptical postmodern sensibility: to approach the idea of God in a radically new way, manifesting another important feature of the robust imagination, what O'Donohue calls the "grace of innocence".

The "grace of innocence" refers to the notion that the imagination does not easily give way to the blast of facts, detached analysis and explanations that constitute the received wisdom about a particular thing or experience. It is not persuaded by that which is considered settled, finished, fixed, or framed by authoritative knowledge and authoritative figures. Rather, the imagination believes, as it were, that there is "more" than meets the eye, there are "secret worlds" and "hidden treasures"—similar to what Levinas calls otherness—concealed in the simplest and clearest things if one only, as the Buddhists say, mindfully engages the world, develops the mental skill of attentiveness and emotional openness to one's moment-to-moment awareness of what one is experiencing. For the robust imaginer, reality is not closed, but continuously offers new possibilities and hope, especially for self-transformation and self-transcendence. According to O'Donohue, "the imagination is the faculty that bridges, co-presents, and co-articulates the visible and invisible" (1997, p. 51), it "creates and constructs your depth experience" (*ibid.*, p. 95).

The relevance of all of this to a person's searching and relating to God, at least as I have framed the discussion, is fairly straightforward. Hard-wired into the human condition, says the great religious scholar Huston Smith, is a yearning for "more" than the world of everyday experience can satisfy. Friedrich Hölderlin, the German lyric poet, made a similar observation, "No action, no thought can reach the extent of your desire. That is the glory of man, that nothing suffices" (Abrams, 1971, p. 216). However, continues Smith, the reality that often inspires and satisfies the human desire for "more", and for self-transcendence, is God, regardless of the label that is used. In short, "the human heart is always drawn to the beyond". As we humans tend to comport ourselves in terms of the future, we are "leaning forward into the future", says O'Donohue. The imagination is the organ of fresh perception for discerning manifestations of the "more" and the "beyond" that we associate with God, at least for those who are spiritually awakened, who are lodged in a religious vision.

For O'Donohue, a related aspect of the imagination is that it has a "passion for freedom". The nature of the imagination is to press ahead beyond the usual frontiers, that is, it wants to roam freely beyond the well-travelled borders, without using the usual maps of experience and understanding to make sense of things. In the essay "Fate", Emerson says that "the revelation of thought [i.e., the imagination] takes man out of servitude into freedom". Moreover, the imagination paradoxically waits to be surprised, for it knows that there is something about the unforeseen and unanticipated that powerfully touches us, just as it provides insights into what really matters. Thus, the robust imaginer and the God-seeker, as I have described him, have much in common. Both want to engage the world with a "dishabituated eye" (Abrams, 1971, p. 384), "defamiliarizing the familiar" (*ibid.*, p. 379) in order to better apprehend the wonders of ordinary life or, in religious language, to apprehend the glory of God. It is, in part, this inner readiness to be intrigued, surprised, and "disrupted" by the otherness and strangeness of people, the animal–organic and the inorganic, that is a distinguishing feature of the robust imaginer and God-seeker.

The robust use of the imagination also provides us with a renewed sense of youthfulness, especially playfulness of spirit, a necessary quality for engaging God as I have conceived him. O'Donohue aptly quotes the German mystic Meister Eckhart to make this point: "Time makes us old, but eternity makes us young".

The point is that it is through the infinite- and eternity-seeking nature of the imagination that one does not surrender to the deadening routine and predictability that make up so much of life, especially as one gets older. Rather, the robust imaginer is enlivened through his playful imaginative use of his mind and heart and, by doing so, reclaims the depth and intensity of experience, as well as the "urgency, restlessness, and passion", "the wildness of heart", most frequently associated with youth. Psychoanalyst Winnicott famously located this imaginative capacity in a magical realm he called "transitional space", the psychic place where a young child uses a "transitional object", like a loved doll or piece of cloth, as a way of being midway between himself and his mother in the service of separating from her and further individuating, yet still being connected to her: "it is within the space between inner and outer world, which is also the space between people—the transitional space—that intimate relationships and creativity occur" (1971, p. 82). Religion (and art and philosophy), for example, represents an adult form of this imaginative dwelling in transitional space; call it the sacred, and the playful use of transitional objects, call it God or tradition. Such a creative use of the imagination, at its best, allows the spiritually inclined to be able to relate to God as a source of deepening personal growth and development, enlivening, and interconnectedness to people, animals, and things.

Finally, the robust imaginer, like the God-seeker, is open to what in religious language is called "revelation". By revelation, I do not only mean the showing of divine will or truth, as the religious usually characterize it. I also mean the disclosure, especially the surprising disclosure, of something previously hidden or secret, often in one's everyday life, that is judged as extremely valuable and good. As theologian Tillich noted, life-altering existential questions, especially in the theological context, are asked on the basis of "ultimate concern", and they are best answered through revelation. The imagination is the psychic vehicle for receiving such revelations, and it usually does so, says O'Donohue, not in a flash, as popular culture would have it. Rather, he says, the imagination gently coaxes us into new situations, new questions, and new possibilities, more analogous to how one looks at a beautiful painting than a dramatic unfolding, though that, too, can be part of revelation. As we look at the painting, as we gradually engage its otherness, its loveliness and splendour emerge. The same gradual process often characterizes the love relation, whether to a person or to God. As we gradually engage the Other, her summoning nature, her mysterious layering and deep presence moves us, just as her beauty of spirit, mind, and body captivates us. The imagination, thus, often operates according to a principle of suggestiveness and insinuation, even seduction, and it is those features that are perfectly in synchronization with the slow but sure way that God reveals Himself to those who are attentive to such signs. Perhaps one of the most inspired and inspiring points of entry to sense God's presence is an encounter with the beauty, power, and sublimity of Nature. It is to this subject that we now turn.

Nature as God's signature

"I frequently tramped eight or ten miles through the deepest snow to keep an appointment with a beech-tree, or a yellow birch or an old acquaintance among the pines", says Thoreau in *Walden*. Indeed, the incredibly moving, inspiring, sensuous nature of physical beauty, be it a sunset, a vast ocean or towering mountain, two squirrels at play, or, for that matter, a strikingly beautiful woman or man, tends instantly to transport us to a different dimension of the spirit. This new "soul-space" crashes through the "barriers of persona and egoism" (O'Donohue, 2004, p. 10), and opens us up to the intimate otherness of Mother Nature through a radical disordering and disruption of the senses. In the mind and heart of the God-seeker, and for many who are spiritually inclined, the beauty of nature represents an act of "divine condescension", an expression of His infinite love for mankind. In this view, continues Abrams, nature is one of the two key symbol-systems (the other being Scripture) that, through the imagination, allow us to experience a glimpse of eternity, of Divine Presence. It is precisely the developed capacity for such "perceptual transvaluations" and "imaginative seeing" (Abrams, 1971, pp. 400–401)—"to see a world in a Grain of Sand, And a Heaven in a wild flower, Hold Infinity in the palm of your hand, And eternity in an hour" (*ibid.*, pp. 390–391)—that is essential to engage the infinite in Nature, a transient reflection of the "mysterious Presence" we associate with God (*ibid.*, p. 139).

Freud, the secularist, in his short essay "On transience" (1916a), makes a similar observation when he writes: "As regards the beauty of Nature, each time it is destroyed by winter it comes again next year, so that in relation to the length of our lives it can in fact be regarded as eternal" (p. 305).

Long before the just-quoted, well-known poem by William Blake, the ancient religious traditions were affirming that beauty, especially in Nature, is an expression of God's perfection, generosity, and goodness. For example, both in the Hebrew Bible (e.g., the sublime poetry of the Psalms) and the Talmud, there is an adoring love of beauty. In fact, as Hertz further points out, the ancient Rabbis created a special prayer for when one views an animal or tree and another for looking at the first blossoms of spring. Some of the Rabbis actually "viewed the whole of Creation as a process of unfolding beauty; and spoke of God as the Incomparable Artist" (Hertz, 1960, p. 376). Likewise, as I have pointed out elsewhere (Marcus, 2003, pp. 73–74), Confucius believed that, in the order of things, nature provides not only sustenance for human survival, but also serves as an inspiration for sustainable life. Implicit in the rhythm of nature, such as the changes of the four seasons, are important lessons in perpetual patterns of transformation, that is, regularity, balance, and harmony. In other words, for the Confucian, nature is held in esteem for its bountifulness, generosity, and grandeur in the nurturing environment that it gives us for our survival. Its awesome presence allows us to appreciate the fruitfulness and sanctity of our earthly "home". This sense of nature as home enables the Confucian to find ultimate meaning in ordinary, everyday human existence, to cultivate a sense of inner serenity and unity with nature, that is, a regularized, balanced, and harmonious lifestyle, and to view what some religions view as secular or profane as sacred. Such a view of nature, in which it is viewed with great respect, reverence, and gratitude, reflects the cosmic connectedness that, in part, constitutes the spiritual dimension to Confucian thought.

Finally, Chuang Tzu, the Taoist philosopher, equated the Tao with Nature, in both its spontaneity and its constant flux, each thing developing according to its own nature, in its own way and time. The Tao, Burton Watson continues, is not God, a prime mover, directing this process of constant change; it is, rather, the "totality of existence" that "embraces all forms of being, all life" (*ibid.*, p. 83). Though things appear to develop from simple to higher life, says Farzeen Baldrian, and finally to humans, ultimately we, too, return to simple stuff, thus concluding the cycle of change. By identifying with the vital rhythms of Nature, the individual participates in the infinity of the universe. His or her life is no longer strictly limited by biology and social context because he or she is now symbiotically related to the cosmos. He or she has fused with the Tao (*ibid.*). Nature, in other words, for most ancient religious traditions, especially Western ones, can be viewed as "a direct expression of the divine imagination" (O'Donohue, 1994, p. 50) that "touches human presence" in a uniquely illuminating, uplifting and instructive way (*ibid.*, p. 50, 76).

As the above comments indicate, Nature has always been a way for man to engage what we in the West often call God or Divine Presence, or its equivalent notion in the East, mainly because it provides a sense of self-transformation and self-transcendence, but in an extremely emotionally compelling and satisfying manner. Indeed, there is something to the psychoanalytic insight that the inspiring, if not sublime, experience of Mother Nature is roughly equivalent to the return to the bliss associated deep within our unconscious of the gentle and loving embrace of our real or imagined mother or care-giver. It is quite plausible that what makes Mother Nature so summoning is that one feels the comforting M[Other] inside you, this being analogous to the gentle, kind, intimate "first Other of the universe", God (*ibid.*, p. 12). It is this beautiful and exquisite "luminosity" and intensity of Her Presence, a "mother-presence" (*ibid.*, p. 15), that evokes the "primal inner peace" and gentle intimacy that we so much associate with Nature—and God—at her numinous best (*ibid.*, p. 37). As psychoanalyst Rycroft (1968) points out, Romain Rolland, one of Freud's early admirers, first described this mystical, cosmic sentiment, the authentic origin of the religious impulse, as "oceanic". The oceanic, thought Freud, is a revival of "the experience of the infant at the breast before he has learned to distinguish his ego from the external world" (*ibid.*, p. 101). It is perhaps this sublimated experience, with its subtle erotically tinged charge, that best accounts for "the profound and numinous presence of Nature", imaginatively experienced as a form of Divine Presence (*ibid.*, p. 96). For many people, it is precisely through this imaginative sympathy with Nature that they feel most in vibrant and resonant contact with God.

Thus far, we have described the possibility of access to God, or at least a sense of His momentary presence, in terms of the imaginative capacity to infuse the infinite into the finite and the eternal into the temporal through the creative and inspired embrace of beauty in Nature. In this view, God's gift to humanity centrally includes the faculty of imagination that can transiently intuit a real, living, though invisible, God "out there", a deep, enlivening presence that matters deeply to the spiritual pilgrim, that is profoundly self-transformative and self-transcendent, and whose wonderful otherness is revealed, in part, through the loveliness of Mother Nature. In one of his letters, Keats writes that "I feel more and more every day, as my imagination strengthens, that I do not live in this world alone but in a thousand worlds" (O'Donohue, 2004, p. 9).

As should be obvious to the reader, my "take" on the God-search and God-experience is heavily rooted in an analogy between religion and poetry, in that they both require a robust, transfiguring imagination in order to make contact with their profoundly transformative beauty that is often associated with Divine Presence. However, the perception of beauty, including the beauty of Nature as I have described it, does not necessarily correlate with Goodness, especially as Levinas defines it, that is, as being for the Other. Indeed, Tolstoy noted in *The Kreutzer Sonata* that "it is amazing how complete [is] the delusion that beauty is goodness". One just has to think of the violent side of Nature, like Hurricane Katrina, to realize that beauteous Mother Nature can be unbelievably ugly in her cruelty. Likewise, the perception of beauty, with its summoning appeal, can be ill-conceived and self-destructive. Think of the Greek sirens, whose lovely song had alluring appeal with disastrous effects for the sailors who heeded its call. That being said, beauty and goodness are often co-mingled, including in the ethical domain (indeed, there is something beautifully good about a fireman who rushes into a burning house and rescues a whimpering, nearly-asphyxiated baby), but they need not be, and sometimes confusing superficial beauty for something judged as truly desirable and good can be lethal to the soul, if not the body.

Thus, if the imagination can be faulty and corrupt, if it can confuse and distort that which is truly infinitely and eternally

Good, just as Mother Nature, so often gentle and lovely, can be terribly cruel, then we need to have a more secure basis for our God-conception, God-search, and God-experience. While establishing such a relatively secure basis is a tremendously philosophically and psychologically complex task, I want at least to point to what I think is perhaps the most creative, subversive, and life-affirming ground on which to meet God, which is love, conceived by Levinas as responsibility for the Other, especially before oneself. Indeed, "love is the threshold where divine and human presence ebb and flow into each other" (O'Donohue, 1997, p. 15). It is this respectful interflow of "otherness and intimacy" that is the ultimate context for embracing the infinite and eternal here on earth, to achieve a kind of "spiritual, soulful self-presence" (*ibid.*, p. 182), what the secularist might simply call deep and abiding peace of mind.

The "royal road" to God: goodness

"I think that God has no meaning outside the search for God", Levinas famously wrote in *Of God Who Comes to Mind* (1998c, p. 95). As I have pointed out elsewhere (Marcus, 2008), what Levinas was getting at is that God is otherwise than being and beyond essence, that is, beyond intellectual–emotional grasp or apprehension using our familiar modes of thought, feeling, and perceiving. Rather, as Levinas says, his focus is on a different question: "What is it to have become conscious of God?" He proposed to explore "the possibility—or even the fact—of understanding the word as a significant word" (1998c, p. xi). His concern, he says, is to describe "the phenomenological 'circumstances', the 'staging' surrounding what gets described in the abstract" (*ibid.*). In other words, for Levinas, the conventional philosophical, theological, and psychological ways of speaking about God are inadequate, and thus he prefers to speak of "to-God" (1998a, pp. 174–175). By "to-God" he means that God is "surrendered" to, "opened up" to, "approached", or "addressed", but never actually directly encountered or arrived at (Hutchens, 2004, p. 118; Davis, 1996, p. 98). This is because God is not a substance or essence and has no independent existence, at least as we conventionally conceive Him (Davis, 1996, p. 98). God is, thus, best conceptualized as a direction rather than an end point, a process rather than a result, a mysterious irruption to be pursued, but never possessed. Embracing such a way of looking at God is, in part, what Levinas means when he speaks of a "religion for adults".

For Levinas, God, or at least a trace of the Divine, is co-present—God "comes to mind"— as one approaches the Other in responsibility, that is, in love, goodness, and justice. As Levinas says, "Through my relation to the Other, I am in touch with God"; "The dimension of the divine opens forth from the human face [i.e., the human personality]". The pragmatic implication of this claim was stated clearly by Levinas, who was mainly interested in understanding what constitutes holiness in real life: when "the concern for the other breaches concern for the self. This is what I call holiness. Our humanity consists in being able to recognize the priority of the other".

What Levinas is getting at is a deep point that has been profoundly elaborated by all of the major ancient religious traditions, which is, "we have a sacred responsibility to encourage and illuminate all that is inherently good and special in each other" (O'Donohue, 2004, p. 172). It is through selfless service to the Other that one is most authentically doing God's work, and by doing so—and this is not the reason for doing selfless service, says Levinas—one is often blessed by a sense of Divine love and compassion, psychologically experienced as living in an ethically caring universe, perhaps the surest basis for relative peace of mind. Stated in more conventional psychological, though paradoxical, terms, it is through living a life of responsibility for the Other before oneself, that is, through an all-embracing altruistic outlook and behaviour, that one can derive a greater sense of "spiritual soulful self-presence". Such a way of being in the world is often correlated both with a greater acceptance of one's otherness—including one's inevitable woundedness and self-damage, and feeling more in harmony with ourselves and the world, with "primal Eros" (*ibid.*, p. 232), what is called, by health psychologists, "well-being", "optimal functioning", and/or "happiness".

As I have written a chapter on the adult-to-adult love relationship, I want here to simply to highlight in what way being for the Other possibly points to God, at least for the person who is spiritually inclined. In short, all acts of kindness and goodness, the lived essence of Levinas's philosophy, puts us in contact with a different, deeper dimension of being, characterized by a heightened sense of immediacy and presence, and intimacy and warmth, that *feels* as if we have become connected to something utterly beyond ourselves, a spiritual force, presence, or being, what believers call God. In other words, to the believer, to paraphrase Heschel, the spiritual quest for the Divine is one in which both man is in search of God and God is in search of man, with their meeting place the space of love, personified by kindness and goodness in one's outlook and behaviour towards others, human, animal–organic, and inorganic. O'Donohue makes a similar point:

> Rather than trying to set out like some isolated cosmonaut in search of God, maybe the secret is to let God find you. Instead of endeavoring to reach out in order to first find God, you realize you are now within the matrix and the adventure is the discovering of utterly new and unspoken dimensions of the inexhaustible divine. [2004, p. 227]

Heschel, the Rabbi, and O'Donohue, the Celtic-inspired spiritualist, are both emphasizing, as does Levinas, that above all else—more than through creating great thoughts or beautiful ideas, works of art, or embracing the loveliness of Nature—it is everyday acts of loving kindness that bring one in imaginative touch with the lyrical, if not sublime, presence of God, in others, in the world, and in oneself. Goodness is not only good for the Other, it almost always resonates in the doer with a non-prideful feeling of being good, too. This is another way of experiencing God's graciousness, in gratitude.

Love, and all acts of kindness, especially on an everyday basis, say with one's spouse or significant other (or, even more so, towards a stranger), is not simply an act of a benign will, it also requires a robust imagination. As American journalist Henry Louis Mencken quipped, "Love is the triumph of imagination over intelligence". This daily capacity to re-imagine the Other in a loving light, says Freud, is related to the ability to idealize the Other, to think or represent her as being perfect, ignoring any perfections that exist or may exist in reality. Without this capacity to idealize, in religious terms, to perceive what is sacred in the Other, it would be nearly impossible to live with someone day in and day out without being bored or seriously tainted by ambivalence and a wide range of negative affects. Voltaire says that "Love is a canvas furnished by nature and embroidered by imagination". Love, in other words, is the continuous renewal of the lyrical imagination within and between two people.

Love also requires a finely tuned empathy for the Other—the ability to identify and understand another person's feelings or difficulties, and this capacity requires a developed imaginative faculty. In order to be accurately empathic, one needs to be able to imagine what the Other feels and thinks, her subjective experience, through the mindful using of one's own subjective experience as a guide. To accomplish all of this in a way that is satisfying to the Other requires paying great creative attention to, and care of, the inner world of the Other, as well as to one's own internal experience. Put simply, it is through the "contemplative imagination" (O'Donohue, 2004, p. 143) that one can discern and engage the "rich strangeness" (*ibid*., p. 144) of the Other "and the intimate strangeness of the self" (*ibid*., p. 227), this being the best of spirituality and God-seeking through the Other. Such an "awakening of real presence", a kind of "eternal surge, a total quickening" (*ibid*., p. 226), is invoked in all acts of love and goodness.

Overcoming the impediments to meeting the Divine

The comportment to the world that I am describing, one that is orientated "to-God", as Levinas called it, that is also perhaps most likely to evoke the self-transformational and self-transcendent sense of God's presence, especially the ethical deepening and expansion that it entails, involves an awareness that the infinite and the eternal lie all about us. The "trick" to embracing such a sensibility is the capacity to pierce "through the perceptual illusions"—rooted in the dulling and muting cognitive and emotional ways of seeing and feeling, the restrictive conventional and familiar ways of being in the world—that foreclose our capacity to engage graciously and reverentially the sacred otherness of God, Nature and the Other (Abrams, 1974, p. 132). In this view, it is the imagination that is key to sensing this "divine Otherness" and "divine presence" that is the basis for such a sanctified, soul-transforming engagement with the Other (O'Donohue, 2004, pp. 242–243). Moreover, as I have suggested, it is by means of a robust imagination that one can reside more securely, deeply, and widely in the ethical realm of being for the Other, of living a life that is "for the Good, from the Good, in the Good, and to the Good" (Abrams, 1971, p. 150).

In this context, one should never forget what Picasso said, "Everything you can imagine is real". This means that, to the extent that one can refine, deepen, and enlarge one's imagination, especially one's ethical imagination—that the other's material needs are my spiritual needs, to paraphrase one of Levinas's favourite Rabbis, Israel Salanter—then one will think, feel, and, most importantly, act in a way that is more in keeping with goodness and, perhaps, derive the "blessed self-forgetfulness" and joy associated with nearness to God that all believers long for. Self-forgetfulness has two meanings here: putting other's needs before oneself, and the individual's freedom from destructive self-obsession, such as we see in anxiety and depressive disorders and, of course, in narcissistic conditions. In fact, when one is fully other-directed and other-regarding, one is released from the burden of one's own existence, from one's own pain, at least during the time of our service, and this benefit of being for the Other should not be underrated.

To claim that to live the Good life, the "to-God" life as described above, is easy, is, of course, a huge understatement. To quote Picasso again, "to see things in a new way, that is really difficult". In other words, it is not a simple thing to reconfigure who one is, to change one's conventional ways of thinking, feeling, and seeing, let alone acting, so as to better perceive and personify goodness in one's everyday life. As I have emphasized throughout this book, human selfishness, extreme self-interest, ego consciousness, and excessive narcissism are the main obstacles for living a life that is animated by love and responsibility for the Other. While both Eastern and Western writers have observed that a loveless life is toxic to the soul: "Not loving is but a long dying", said the famous emperor of the Han Dynasty, Wu Ti, and Dostoevsky repeatedly says in *Notes from the Underground*, "Hell is the place where a person lives who is unable to love", the fact is that the self-centric, "for oneself" way of being in the world, painful and self-imprisoning as it is, does not easily give way to being for the Other, as psychoanalysts have aptly shown. Fear, among other debilitating and complex affects, often gets in the way.

In his paper "On transience" (1916a), Freud perceptively put his finger on one often overlooked aspect of this fear of loving the Other, whether the Other be human, Nature, or God. Writing in the context of a walk with two friends, one a poet, Freud notes that they could not wholeheartedly appreciate the beauty of the "smiling" countryside. Said Freud: "The poet admired the beauty of the scene around us but felt no joy in it". Freud then speculates,

> What spoilt their enjoyment of beauty must have been a revolt in their minds against mourning. The idea that all this beauty was transient was giving these two sensitive minds a foretaste of mourning over its decease; and, since the mind instinctively recoils from anything that is painful, they felt their enjoyment of beauty interfered with by thoughts of transience. [*ibid.*, p. 306]

In other words, one of the impediments to engaging God, in whatever form, is the awareness that, in a certain sense, it is a limited engagement; His felt presence is fleeting, as any honest believer will tell you, and we have to mourn His loss, time and again. For some, this is simply too painful, and so they do not engage God, just as others do not enter into a love relation, or others open themselves up to the disclosures of Nature's beauty. The idea of the inevitable loss of connection and communion with the Other is so troubling, so utterly overwhelming, that they close themselves off from any such potential traumatic loss by never letting themselves be awakened to God in the first place. Such a defensive, closed-off way of being robs life of much of its aliveness, depth, and fun.

As for the problem of developing a more open, inclusive, interdependent non-self-centred subjectivity regulated mainly by goodness, the kind of subjectivity that I am suggesting is the most fertile breeding ground for letting a trace of God's presence into one's everyday life. I want to mention briefly at least three interdependent qualities of mind and heart that seem essential: reverence, humility, and graciousness. Needless to say, there is much more to all of this than space permits me to elaborate (O'Donohue, 2004, p. 31).

While I have emphasized that there will always be a disconnect "between man['s] infinite reach and his finite grasp" (Abrams, 1971, p. 216), it is the cultivation of reverence, feelings of deep respect and devotion before the mystery of life that seems crucial. As Albert Schweitzer wrote, "reverence for life affords me my fundamental principle of morality, namely, that good consists in maintaining, assisting and enhancing life and that to destroy, to harm, or to hinder life is evil . . . Ethics is nothing else than reverence for life". It is through a reverential attitude that the Other's dignity and beauty emerge, it being rooted in a mindfulness that one is always in the presence of the sacred, whether one's point of entry is the person, Nature, or another God-infused portal. As the ancient Taoist philosopher, Chuang Tzu, said, the Tao (defined by one scholar as "the unique source of the universe that determines all things") is even "in the piss and shit". God is, in other words, at least psychologically speaking, wherever one imagines he is, and if this outlook is suffused with ethicality as I, following Levinas, have described it, it is real, or "real enough" to make a profound difference in how one lives one's life.

Needless to say, humility, the quality of being respectful and modest, is often co-present when one is properly reverential in one's comportment. Narcissism, selfishness, pride, and the like utterly close off one's access "to God", for, by their very nature, they obscure the sacred otherness of the person, the beauty of nature, and divine otherness. Put more simply, when one is utterly wrapped up in oneself, one is not easily captivated by anyone or anything else (let alone able to feel responsible for them), except perhaps as objects to use for self-aggrandizement, self-nourishment, and other forms of need satisfaction. Humility, as I have written elsewhere, is the moral virtue that prevents a person from seeking gratification of unreasonable and unrealistic desires for self-aggrandizement and self-affirmation, those prideful desires being the basis of much unhappiness. By having a sense of both God's infinite love and power and one's ultimate lack of self-sufficiency and powerlessness in the universe, we are more likely to have reasonable expectations for our lives (Marcus, 2003, p. 149).

Finally, we come to graciousness, that which Levinas calls goodness or kindness, but also includes courtesy and politeness. For Levinas, it is goodness that is the royal road "to God", for it is through the everyday concern for the Other—as he famously says, like opening the door and saying, "After you"—that most depicts what it means to have internalized being for the Other before oneself, and thus perhaps to sense for a fleeting moment the "sublime space where God holds us, a space of infinite graciousness where we are cherished and loved". Our graciousness to others evokes God's graciousness, the former being a derivative of the latter in the mind and heart of the believer. It is in this sublime space, continues O'Donohue, that "the soul comes to bathe in the stream of mercy", experienced as being cared about by God (2004, pp. 240–241). Indeed, while Levinas was not prone to the lyrical mystical-sounding language O'Donohue uses, he makes a similar point when he writes, "It is [in] the human face that . . . *the trace of God is manifested, and the light of revelation inundates the universe"* (original italics) (1996b, p. 95).

Following Levinas, God thus appears to me in the manner of a numinous trace that is the face of the Other, that is, the "saintliness of God" is best accessed and affirmed in responsibility for the Other, through deeds of love and justice. As Rabbi Hertz points out, for the ancient Rabbis, "while man cannot imitate God's infinity, omnipotence or eternity . . . he can know His 'goodness' . . . Man is never nearer to the Divine than in his compassionate moments" (1960, p. 363). Levinas is deeply lodged in the best of all the great religious traditions and spiritualities that recognize that the "Good life" is one that is bathed in goodness, in a way of being in the world personified by its reverence for life, especially its mystery, humility, and graciousness, among other classical moral virtues. As Aristotle said in the *Nichomachean Ethics,* sounding a bit like Levinas, "The good has been well said to be that at which all things aim". Mother Teresa, religiously ambivalent as she apparently was, aptly tells us, especially to the believer, what this means in our everyday quest for the Good Life, "Let every action of mine be something beautiful for God".

GLOSSARY

The short glossary below is meant to help the uninitiated reader of Levinas to better grasp his extremely hard going, specialized terminology. Each entry starts with a short orientating quote from Levinas, followed by a few sentences to help clarify what I think Levinas was getting at, especially as it relates to how the term is used in my book. For those of you who want to read Levinas, I would start with two books of interviews, *Ethics and Infinity: Conversations with Philippe Nemo* (1985) and *Is It Righteous To Be? Interviews with Emmanuel Levinas* (2001a). From there you can tackle his more demanding texts, such as his two masterpieces, *Totality and Infinity: An Essay on Exteriority* (1969), and *Otherwise Than Being: Or Beyond Essence* (1998b). As for good introductory secondary sources, some of the best are Colin Davis's *Levinas, An Introduction* (1996), Benjamin C. Hutchens' *Levinas: A Guide for the Perplexed* (2004), Peter Atterton and Matthew Calarco's *On Levinas* (2005), and Edith Wyschogrod's *Emmanuel Levinas: The Problem of Ethical Metaphysics* (2nd edition) (2000). If the reader is interested in the Levinas/psychoanalysis connection, my *Being For The Other. Emmanuel Levinas, Ethical Living and Psychoanalysis*, is a good book to start with. I have liberally relied on Atterton and Calarco's and Wyschogrod's glossaries to help prepare my own.

Alterity: "The absolutely other is the Other." Alterity is equivalent to otherness, that which is not myself.

Ethics: ". . . ethics is no longer a simple moralism of rules which decree what is virtuous. It is the original awakening of an I responsible for the other; the accession of my person to the uniqueness of the I called and elected to responsibility for the other." Ethics is the putting into question of the "I" by the Other, that is, the upsurge of self-awareness that the Other is "out there" and needs our help, and who thus summons us to responsibility for the Other.

Face: "The face has turned to me—and this is its very nudity. It is by itself and not by reference to a system . . . The relation with the face is not an object-cognition [it is not a thought or perception as conventionally understood] . . . The nakedness of the face is destituteness. To recognize the Other is to recognize a hunger. To recognize the Other is to give." Says Wyschogrod, the face, roughly equivalent to the personality, "is the source of revelation of the other who cannot be encompassed in cognition [cannot be thematized, pinned down, made into a generality, an abstract totality, as in psychology and sociology for example]. It calls separated being, egoity, the self into question" (i.e., the face irresistibly grabs our attention, it troubles us, and thus summons us to responsibility for the Other).

Good: "Goodness consists in taking up a position such that the Other counts more than myself." Goodness is thus radical altruism, personified in the lives of saints and *tzadikim* (the Hebrew word for righteous people).

Hostage: "To be oneself, the state of being a hostage, is always to have one degree of responsibility, the responsibility for the responsibility of the other . . . I exist through the other and for the other, but without this being alienation; I am inspired." To be a hostage means that human subjectivity, the self, humanity, is, first and foremost, characterized by responsibility for the Other. Responsibility is not derivative of anything else, as in psychoanalytic conceptions (e.g., instinct or object relations, etc.), it is the bedrock of existence.

Other: "The absolutely other is the Other"; "The Other . . . is what I am not." Says Wyschogrod, the term "Other" is "reserved for the special alterity [otherness] belonging to other persons who resist reduction to the same [that is, a view of the Other that destroys his uniqueness and individuality]. The Other stands in an asymmetrical relation with oneself. The Other is always higher, commands, is the teacher of the self" [that is, the reasonable material, psychological, and spiritual needs of the Other take precedence over the self].

Responsibility: Responsibility for the Other is "the essential, primary, and fundamental structure of responsibility. . . . I understand responsibility as responsibility for the Other, thus as responsibility for what is not my deed, or for what does not even matter to me; or which precisely does matter to me, is met by me as a face". Responsibility for the Other is not originally chosen, it is the human condition; thus, it cannot be refused (i.e., it is prior to freedom). Moreover, it is non-symmetrical, that is, it does not initially seek out reciprocity and it is not transferable. Levinas often cites Dostoyevsky when discussing responsibility, "We are all responsible for all for all men before all, and I more than all the others."

Self: "Perhaps the possibility of a point of the universe where such an overflow of responsibility is produced ultimately defines the I"; "The self is *sub-jectum*; it is under the weight of the universe, responsible for everything". Levinas's formulation of the self thus challenges all psychoanalytic theories—Freud, Klein, Erikson, Kohut, and Lacan, for example, that assume that man is, first and foremost, egocentric and self-centric in outlook and behaviour.

Totality: "Yet totality should not leave anything outside." Totalization is the tendency to reduce the Other to a rationally intelligible, thematizable and thus manipulable entity. According to Wyschogrod, such a "view of the whole," undermines if not destroys the otherness of the Other (his uniqueness and individuality), and is thus "a primal act of violence." The opposite tendency to totalization Levinas calls "infinity"—something outside of and beyond everything, like the Other, ethics, transcendence, and God.

REFERENCES

AARP Magazine (2006). July–August.
Abrams, M. H. (1971). *Natural Supernaturalism: Tradition and Revolution in Romantic Literature*. New York: W. W. Norton.
Alford, C. F. (1998). Melanie Klein and the nature of good and evil. In: P. Marcus & A. Rosenberg (Eds.), *Psychoanalytic Versions of the Human Condition: Philosophies of Life and Their Impact on Practice* (pp. 117–139). New York: New York University Press.
Amato, P., & Patridge, S. (1989). *The New Vegetarians: Promoting Health and Protecting Life*. New York: Plenum Press.
Assoun, P.-L. (2000). *Freud and Nietzsche*, R. L. Collier (Trans.). London: Continuum.
Atterton, P. (2004). Face-to-face with the other animal. In: P. Atterton, M. Calarco, & M. S. Friedman (Eds.), *Levinas and Buber: Dialogue and Difference* (pp. 262–281). Pittsburgh, PA: Duquesne University Press.
Atterton, P., & Calarco, M. (2005). *On Levinas*. Belmont, CA: Thomson Wadsworth.
Auden, W. H. (Ed.) (1966). *The Selected Poetry and Prose of Byron*. New York: The New American Library.
Ayim, M. (1994). Knowledge through the grapevine: gossip as inquiry. In: R. F. Goodman & A. Ben-Ze'ev (Eds.), *Good Gossip* (pp. 85–99). Lawrence, KS: University Press of Kansas.

Balcombe, J. (2006). *The Pleasurable Kingdom: Animals and the Nature of Feeling Good*. New York: Macmillan.

Bass, A. (1998). The question of a weltanschauung and of defense. In: P. Marcus & A. Rosenberg (Eds.), *Psychoanalytic Version of the Human Condition: Philosophies of Life and Their Impact on Practice* (pp. 412–446). New York: New York University Press.

Becker, A. (2006). Pet sounds. *The New York Times Book Review*, 26 March, p. 17; *The Boston Phoenix*, 30 June, p. 6.

Becker, E. (1969). *Angel in Armor: A Post·Freudian Perspective on the Nature of Man*. New York: Braziller.

Bergman, M. S. (1987). *The Anatomy of Loving: The Story of Man's Quest to Know What Love Is*. New York: Fawcett Columbine.

Bickerman, E. (1967). *Four Strange Books of the Bible*. New York: Schocken Books.

Breton, S. (2004). Being God, and the poetics of relation. In: R. Kearney (Ed.), *Debates in Continental Philosophy. Conversations With Contemporary Thinkers* (pp. 126–138). New York: Fordham University Press.

Breuer, J., & Freud, S. (1895d). *Studies on Hysteria*. *S.E.*, *2*: 1–335. London: Hogarth.

Buber, M. (1965). *Between Man and Man*. New York: Macmillan.

Calin, R. (2005). The exception of testimony. In: J. Bloechl & J. L. Kosky (Eds.), *Levinas Studies*, Volume 1 (pp. 73–97). Pittsburgh, PA: Duquesne University Press.

Camus, A. (1991). *The Fall*. New York: Vintage.

Carnes, P. (1989). *Contrary to Love: Helping the Sexual Addict*. Center City, MN: Hazelden Publishers.

Chofetz Chaim (Kagan, Y. M.) (1975). *Guard Your Tongue*. Union City, NJ: Gross Bros.

Cohen, A. (Ed.) (1970). *The Five Megilloth*. London: Soncino Press.

Cohen, M. S. (2000). Personal communication, 12 January.

Cohen, R. A. (2002). Maternal psyche. In: E. E. Gantt & R. N. Williams (Eds.), *Psychology For the Other. Levinas, Ethics and the Practice of Psychology* (pp. 32–64). Pittsburgh, PA: Duquesne University Press.

Cohen, R. A. (2005). Review of Emmanuel Levinas's *On Escape*. *European Journal of Psychotherapy, Counseling and Health*, *7*(1–2): 109–115.

Cohen, R. A. (2007). Personal communication.

Collins, L. (1994). Gossip: a feminist defense. In: R. Goodman & A. Ben-Ze'ev (Eds.), *Good Gossip* (pp. 106–116). Lawrence, KS: University Press of Kansas.

Crenshaw, J. L. (1987). *Ecclesiastes: A Commentary* (Old Testament Library). Philadelphia: Westminster.

Davis, C. (1996). *Levinas: An Introduction*. Cambridge: Polity Press.
Derrida, J. (1999). *Adieu to Emmanuel Levinas*, P.-A. Brault & M. Nass (Trans.). Stanford, CA: Stanford University Press.
Dickey, J. (1970). *Deliverance*. New York: Dell.
Dovidio, J. F., & Penner, L. A. (2001). Helping and altruism. In: G. Fletcher & M. Clark (Eds.). *Blackwell Handbook of Social Psychology Interpersonal Process* (pp. 162–195). Oxford: Blackwell.
Edmundson, M. (2007). Defender of the faith? *New York Times Magazine*, 9 September, Section 4: 15–19.
Eigen, M. (2007). Guilt in an age of psychopathy. *Psychoanalytic Review*, 94(5): October, 727–749.
Eissler, K. (1962). *Leonardo Da Vinci: Psycho-Analytic Notes on the Enigma*. London: The Hogarth Press.
Emler, N. (1994). Gossip, reputation, and social adaptation. In: R. Goodman & A. Ben-Ze'ev (Eds.), *Good Gossip* (pp. 117–138). Lawrence, KS: University Press of Kansas.
Erikson, E. H. (1964). *Insight and Responsibility: Lecture on the Ethical Implications of Psychoanalytic Insight*. New York: W. W. Norton.
Fine, R. (1979). *A History of Psychoanalysis*. New York: Columbia University Press.
Foucault, M. (1989). The ethics of the concern for self as a practice of freedom. In: S. Lotringer (Ed.), *Foucault Live, Collected Interviews, 1961–1984* (pp. 432–449). New York: Semiotext(e).
Fox, M. (1999). *Deep Vegetarianism*. Philadelphia, PA: Temple University Press.
Fraiberg, S. (1980). *Clinical Studies in Infant Mental Health*. New York: Basic Books.
Freud, S. (1905[1904]). On psychotherapy. *S.E.*, *7*: 255–268.
Freud, S. (1905d). *Three Essays on the Theory of Sexuality*. *S.E.*, *7*: 125–245. London: Hogarth.
Freud, S. (1910c). *Leonardo Da Vinci and a Memory of his Childhood*. *S.E.*, *11*: 57–137. London: Hogarth.
Freud, S. (1913c). On beginning the treatment. *S.E.*, *12*: 123–144. London: Hogarth.
Freud, S. (1915a). Observations on transference love: further recommendations in the technique of psychoanalysis. *S.E.*, *12*: 157–172. London: Hogarth.
Freud, S. (1916–1917[1915–1917]). Introductory lectures on psychoanalysis. *S.E.*, *16*: 416.
Freud, S. (1916a). On transience. *S.E.*, *14*: 303–308. London. Hogarth.

Freud, S. (1923b). *The Ego and the Id. S.E., 19*: 3–66. London: Hogarth.
Freud, S. (1930a). *Civilization and its Discontents. S.E., 21*: 57–145. London: Hogarth.
Fromm, E. (1956). *The Art of Loving: An Enquiry into the Nature of Love.* New York: Harper Colophon Books.
Fryer, D. R. (2004). *The Intervention of the Other. Ethical Subjectivity in Levinas and Lacan.* New York: Other Press.
Ginsberg, H. L. (1969). *The Five Megilloth and Jonah.* Philadelphia, PA: Jewish Publication Society of America.
Gluckman, M. (1963). Gossip and scandal. *Current Anthropology, 4*(3): 307–316.
Goffman, E. (1961). *Asylums.* Garden City, NJ: Anchor Books.
Goodman, R., & Ben-Ze'ev, A. (Eds.) (1994). *Good Gossip.* Lawrence, KS: University Press of Kansas.
Gordis, R. (1951). *Koheleth—The Man and His World.* New York: Jewish Theological Seminary of America.
Greenberg, I. (1977). Cloud of smoke, pillar of fire: Judaism, Christianity, and modernity after the Holocaust. In: E. Fleischner (Ed.), *Auschwitz: Beginning of a New Era? Reflections on the Holocaust* (pp. 7–56). New York: KTAV.
Greenberg, J. R., & Mitchell, S. A. (1983). *Object Relations in Psychoanalytic Theory.* Cambridge: Harvard University Press.
Greer, G. (1972). *The Female Eunuch* (1st edn). New York: Bantam.
Grier, K. C. (2006). *Pets in America: A History.* Chapel Hill, NC: University of North Carolina Press.
Guthrie, D., & Motyer, J. A. (Eds.) (1970). *The New Bible Commentary: Revised* (pp. 570–578). Grand Rapids, MI: Eerdmans Publishing.
Hadot, P. (1997). *Philosophy as a Way of Life.* Oxford: Blackwell.
Hall, C., & Lindzey, G. (1978). *Theories of Personality* (3rd edn). New York: John Wiley.
Hatley, J. (2006). Persecution and expiation: a Talmudic amplification of the enigma of responsibility in Levinas. *Philosophy Today,* Spring, *50*(1): 80–91.
Heilman, S. (1973). *Synagogue Life: A Study in Symbolic Interaction.* Chicago, IL: University of Chicago Press.
Henslin, J. (1995). *Sociology: A Down-to-Earth Approach* (2nd edn). New York: Simon and Schuster, Inc.
Hertz, J. H. (1960). *The Pentateuch and Haftorahs: Hebrew Text, English Translation and Commentary* (2nd edn). London: Soncino Press.
Heschel, A. J. (1955). *God in Search of Man: A Philosophy of Judaism.* New York: Farrar, Straus and Giroux.

Hutchens, B. C. (2004). *Levinas: A Guide For the Perplexed*. New York: Continuum.
Hutter, H. (2006). *Shaping The Future Nietzsche's New Regime of the Soul and Its Ascetic Practices*. Lanham, MD: Lexington Books.
Jacobs, J. (2001). *Choosing Character: Responsibility for Virtue and Vice*. Ithaca, NY: Cornell University Press.
Jaeger, M., Skleder, A., Rind, B., & Rosnow, R. (1994). Gossip, gossipers, gossipees. In: R. Goodman & A. Ben-Ze'ev (Eds.), *Good Gossip* (pp. 154–168). Lawrence, KS: University Press of Kansas.
Kosky, J. (2001). *Levinas and the Philosophy of Religion*. Bloomington, IN: Indiana University Press.
Kunz, G. (1998). *The Paradox of Power and Weakness: Levinas and an Alternative Paradigm for Psychology*. Albany, NY: State University of New York Press.
Leary, M. (2001). The self we know and the self we show: self-esteem, self-presentation, and the maintenance of interpersonal relationships. In: *Blackwell Handbook of Social Psychology Interpersonal Process*, pp. 456–477. Oxford: Blackwell.
Levinas, E. (1969). *Totality and Infinity: an Essay on Exteriority*, A. Lingis (Trans.). Pittsburgh, PA: Duquesne University Press.
Levinas, E. (1985). *Ethics and Infinity: Conversations with Philippe Nemo*, R. A. Cohen (Trans.). Pittsburgh, PA: Duquesne University Press.
Levinas, E. (1987). *Time and the Other*, R. A. Cohen (Trans.). Pittsburgh, PA: Duquesne University Press.
Levinas, E. (1988). *The Provocation of Levinas: Rethinking the Other*, R. Bernasconi & D. Wood (Eds.). London: Routledge.
Levinas, E. (1989a). *Difficult Freedom: Essays on Judaism*, S. Hand (Trans.). Evanston, IL: Northwestern University Press.
Levinas, E. (1989b). There is: existence without existents. In: S. Hand (Ed.), *The Levinas Reader* (pp. 29–36). New York: Routledge Books.
Levinas, E. (1990a). *Difficult Freedom: Essays on Judaism*, S. Hand (Trans.). Baltimore, MD: Johns Hopkins University Press.
Levinas, E. (1990b). *Nine Talmudic Readings*, A. Aronowicz (Trans.). Bloomington, IN: Indiana University Press.
Levinas, E. (1994). *In The Time of the Nations*, M. B. Smith (Trans.). Bloomington, IN: Indiana University Press.
Levinas, E. (1996a). *Basic Philosophical Writings*, R. Bernasconi, S. Critchley, & A. Peperzak (Eds.). Bloomington, IN: Indiana University Press.
Levinas, E. (1996b). *Proper Names*, M. B. Smith (Trans.). Stanford, CA: Stanford University Press.

Levinas, E. (1998a). *Entre Nous: Essays on Thinking-of-the-Other,* M. B. Smith & B. Harshav (Trans.). New York: Columbia University Press.

Levinas, E. (1998b). *Otherwise Than Being: Or Beyond Essence,* A. Lingis (Trans.). Pittsburgh, PA: Duquesne University Press.

Levinas, E. (1998c). *Of God Who Comes To Mind,* B. Bergo (Trans.). Stanford, CA: Stanford University Press.

Levinas, E. (2000a). *God, Death, and Time,* B. Bergo (Trans.). Stanford, CA: Stanford University Press.

Levinas, E. (2000b). *Alterity and Transcendence,* M. B. Smith (Trans.). New York: Columbia University Press.

Levinas, E. (2001a). *Is it Righteous To Be? Interviews with Emmanuel Levinas,* J. Robbins (Ed.). Stanford, CA: Stanford University Press.

Levinas, E. (2001b). *Existence and Existents,* A. Lingis (Trans.). Pittsburgh, PA: Duquesne University Press.

Levinas, E. (2003). *On Escape: De l'évasion,* B. Bergo (Trans.). Stanford, CA: Stanford University Press.

Llewelyn, J. (1995). *Emmanuel Levinas. The Genealogy of Ethics*. New York: Routledge.

Marcus, P. (1999). *Autonomy in the Extreme Situation: Bruno Bettelheim, the Nazi Concentration Camps and the Mass Society*. Westport, CT: Praeger.

Marcus, P. (2003). *Ancient Religious Wisdom, Spirituality and Psychoanalysis*. Westport, CT: Praeger.

Marcus, P. (2008). *Being For the Other: Emmanuel Levinas, Ethical Living and Psychoanalysis*. Milwaukee, WI: Marquette University Press.

May, H. G., & Metzger, B. M. (1973). Ecclesiastes. In: *The New Oxford Annotated Bible With the Apocrypha: Revised Standard Versions*. New York: Oxford University Press.

May, R. (1958). Contributions of existential psychotherapy. In: R. May, E. Angel, & H. Ellenberger (Eds.), *Existence A New Dimension in Psychiatry and Psychology* (pp. 37–91). New York: Clarion Books.

McGuire, W. (Ed.) (1974). *The Freud–Jung Letters: The Correspondence Between Sigmund Freud and C. G. Jung*. Princeton: Princeton University Press.

Meissner, W. W. (2003). *The Ethical Dimension of Psychoanalysis: A Dialogue*. Albany, NY: State University of New York Press.

Meltzer, D. (1978). *The Kleinian Development,* Books I, II and III in one volume. Strath Tay, Perthshire: Clunie Press.

Monte, C. (1980). *Beneath The Mask. An Introduction to Theories of Personality* (2nd edn). New York: Holt, Rinehart and Winston.

Moore, B. E., & Fine, B. D. (Eds.) (1990). *Psychoanalytic Terms and Concepts*. New Haven, CT: The American Psychoanalytic Association and Yale University Press.

Morgan, M. L. (2005). Levinas and Judaism. In: J. Bloechl & J. L. Kosky (Eds.), *Levinas Studies, Volume 1* (pp. 1–17). Pittsburg, PA: Duquesne University Press.

Nemo, P. (1998). *Job and the Excess of Evil*. Pittsburgh, PA: Duquesne University Press.

Nevo, O., Nevo, B., & Derech-Zehavi, A. (1994). The technology to gossip as a psychological disposition: constructing a measure and validating it. In: R. Goodman & A. Ben-Ze'ev (Eds.), *Good Gossip* (pp. 180–189). Lawrence, KS: University Press of Kansas.

O'Connor, N. (1961). Who suffers? In: R. Bernasconi & S. Critchley (Eds.), *Re-Reading Levinas*. Indianapolis, IN: Indiana University Press.

O'Donohue, J. (1997). *Anam Cara; A Book of Celtic Wisdom*. New York: Harper Perennial.

O'Donohue, J. (2004). *Beauty: The Invisible Embrace*. New York: Perennial.

Paine, R. (1967). What is gossip about? An alternative hypothesis. *Man*, *2*(2): 278–285.

Pattison, E. M. (1988). The holocaust as sin: requirements in psychoanalytic theory for human evil and mature morality. In: S. Luel & P. Marcus (Eds.), *Psychoanalytic Reflections on the Holocaust: Selected Essays* (pp. 71–94). New York: University of Denver and KTAV Publishers.

Peli, P. H. (1994). *On Repentance: The Thought and Oral Discourses of Rabbi Joseph B. Soloveitchik*. New York: Paulist Press.

Peperzak, A. (1993). *To The Other: An Introduction to the Philosophy of Emmanuel Levinas*. West Lafayette, IN: Purdue University Press.

Perry, T. A. (1993). *Dialogues with Kohelet: The Book of Ecclesiastes*. University Park, PA: Pennsylvania State University Press.

Person, E. S., Cooper, A. M., & Gabbard, G. O. (Eds.) (2005). *Textbook of Psychoanalysis*. Washington, DC: American Psychiatric Association.

Phillips, A. (1998). Paging Dr. Freud. *New York Times Book Review*, p. 24.

Post, R. (1994). The legal regulation of gossip: backyard chatter and the mass media. In: R. Goodman & A. Ben-Ze'ev (Eds.), *Good Gossip* (pp. 65–71). Lawrence, KS: University Press of Kansas.

Preminger, A. (Ed.) (1965). *Encyclopedia of Poetry and Poetics*. Princeton, NJ: Princeton University Press.

Richard, A., Richards, P. S., & Bergin, A. E. (1997). *A Spiritual Strategy for Counseling and Psychotherapy*. Washington, DC: American Psychological Association.

Robbins, J. (Ed.) (2001). *Is It Righteous To Be? Interviews with Emmanuel Levinas*. Stanford, CA: Stanford University Press.

Rosenbaum, J., & Subrin, M. (1963). The psychology of gossip. *Journal of the American Psychoanalytic Association, 11*: 817–831.

Rubin, J. B. (1996). *Psychotherapy and Buddhism: Toward an Integration*. New York: Plenum Press.

Rycroft, C. (1968). *A Critical Dictionary of Psychoanalysis*. Harmondsworth: Penguin.

Santayana, G. (1998). *The Life of Reason*. Amherst, NY: Prometheus Books.

Sartre, J.-P. (1973). *Qu'est-ce que la literature*. Paris: Flammarion.

Schoeman, F. (1994). Gossip and privacy. In: R. Goodman & A. Ben-Ze'ev (Eds.), *Good Gossip* (pp. 72–82). Lawrence, KS: University Press of Kansas.

Scott, R. B. Y. (Ed.) (1965). *The Anchor Bible: Proverbs. Ecclesiastes*. Garden City, NY: Doubleday.

Shafranske, E. P. (Ed.) (1996). *Religion and the Clinical Practice of Psychology*. Washington, DC: American Psychological Association.

Smith, H. (1979). *Forgotten Truth: The Primordial Tradition*. New York: Harper and Row.

Smith, M. B. (2005). *Toward the Outside: Concepts and Themes in Emmanuel Levinas*. Pittsburgh, PA: Duquesne University Press.

Spencer, C. (2000). *Vegetarianism. A History*. New York: Four Walls Eight Windows.

Spiegelman, W. (2002). *The Lives and Works of the English Romantic Poets*. Chantilly, VA: The Teaching Company (Course Guidebook, Parts 1 and 2).

Stewart, P., & Strathern, A. (2004). *Witchcraft, Sorcery, Rumors, and Gossip*. Cambridge: Cambridge University Press.

Suls, J., & Goodkin, F. (1994). Medical gossip and rumor: their role in the lay referral system. In: R. Goodman & A. Ben-Ze'ev (Eds.), *Good Gossip* (pp. 169–179). Lawrence, KS: University Press of Kansas.

Tallon, A. (2007). Can Levinas's ethical metaphysics contribute to psychoanalysis? The case for and against. *Psychoanalytic Review, 94*(4): 657–680.

Target, M. (2006). Attachment theory and research. In: E. S. Person, A. M. Cooper & G. O. Gabbard (Eds.), *Textbook of Psychoanalysis* (pp. 159–172). Washington, DC: American Psychiatric Association.

Taylor, G. (1994). Gossip as moral talk. In: R. Goodman & A. Ben-Ze'ev (Eds.), *Good Gossip* (pp. 34–46). Lawrence, KS: University Press of Kansas.

The Week (2007a). Generation Y: it's all about me. *7*(301): 19.

The Week (2007b). Mother Teresa: the faith that faltered. *7*(327): 19.

Todd, S. (2003). *Learning from the Other*. Albany, NY: State University of New York Press.

Wallwork, E. (2005). Ethics in psychoanalysis. In: E. S. Person, A. M. Cooper & G. O. Gabbard (Eds.), *Textbook of Psychoanalysis* (pp. 281–297). Washington DC: American Psychiatric Association.

Weinstein, F. (1990). *History and Theory After the Fall: An Essay on Interpretation*. Chicago, IL: University of Chicago Press.

Weinstein, A. (1998). *Classics of American Literature, Part 7* (pp. 23–29). Chantilly, VA: The Teaching Company. Course Guidebook.

Williams, R. N. (2007). Levinas and psychoanalysis: the radical turn outward and upward. *Psychoanalytic Review*, *94*(4): 681–703, August.

Winnicott, D. W. (1971). *Playing and Reality*. New York: Basic Books.

www.SixWise.com (2009). Gossip: it can devastate, but here's how it can also be beneficial.

Wyschogrod, E. (2000). *Emmanuel Levinas. The Problem of Ethical Metaphysics* (2nd edn). New York: Fordham University Press.

Young-Bruehl, E. (1988). The biographer's empathy with her subject. In: *Subject to Biography: Psychoanalysis, Feminism, and Writing Women's Lives*. Cambridge, CT: Harvard University Press.

Zlotowitz, M. (1996). *Koheles. Ecclesiastes. A New Translation With a Commentary Anthologized From Talmudic, Midrashic and Rabbinic Sources*. New York: Mesorah.

INDEX

For Product Safety Concerns and Information please contact our EU representative GPSR@taylorandfrancis.com
Taylor & Francis Verlag GmbH, Kaufingerstraße 24, 80331 München, Germany

www.ingramcontent.com/pod-product-compliance
Ingram Content Group UK Ltd.
Pitfield, Milton Keynes, MK11 3LW, UK
UKHW022203190926
475702UK00003B/170

* 9 7 8 0 3 6 7 1 0 6 4 4 7 *